HERE'S WHAT BUSY MOMS LOVE ABOUT

The Moms' Guide to Meal Makeovers:

"Janice and Liz are able to simplify all the mixed messages from the media and translate them into simple, healthy, and creative recipes. I collect many cookbook, but this one I'll enjoy giving to my friends and know that it will be used over and over again. I'll enjoy using it with my daughters, too, as they are now learning to cook themselves!"

—Maureen P., mother of two

"I have been struggling for years to provide good nutrition to picky and opinonated eaters; the strategies Liz and Janice offer are inspiring, totally realistic, and doable. I love their positive suggestions for how to approach this; the concept of taking my kids' favorite 'C' meals and reengineering them slightly to transform them to nutritional but enjoyable 'B+' is empowering. For years I have fallen into the trap of telling my kids why they have to eat certain foods—it is no surprise that they do not want to eat them. With the Makeover Moms' strategies, I believe I can convince my pickiest eater that vegetables actually are delicious and fun to eat!"

—Robin L., mother of two

"I seem to have found something for everyone!! One of the greatest things about this cookbook is that the recipes contain ingredients that I would normally have on my shelf. Far too often when I try new recipes I have to buy ingredients that I use once and that sit on my shelf until the next time that I make that same dish—if there is a next time! If I already have the ingredients, I am more apt to try new recipes. So I know that I will be trying many more of the recipes from your cookbook!"

—Cheryl H., mother of three

"As a mother of four children ranging in ages from three to eleven, life sometimes gets in the way of good nutrition. Because of that I especially liked the 'Moms' Best of Bunch' feature. Many times I have found myself staring at the grocery shelves full of hot dogs trying to find just one that has SOME nutritional value. The 'Best of the Bunch' suggestions will be a great resource to help me keep some quick dinner options on hand without completely abandoning my nutritional standards."

—Sue C., mother of four

"Having three teenage children with very busy schedules, this book has been a tremendous help already. Not only are the meals healthy and easy to prepare, but my children enjoy cooking them as well. My oldest daughter leaves for college next year, and I'm sure she'll take many of these recipes with her."

—Lori H., mother of three

"I felt like the world was working against me when it came to keeping my family healthy. Between questionable school lunches, so many sugary celebrations for kids, and supermarket aisle upon aisle of confusing, even misleading food labels, I was losing the battle. *Moms' Guide to Meal Makeovers* was a breakthrough book for me. Finally, the nutrition information I needed with realistic strategies and recipes to fit it into my family's way of life. Phew!

"Liz and Janice have done a tremendous amount of work sifting through all there is to know about nutrition, studying product labels and testing recipes to bring us what we moms need to know about feeding our families and no more! With name-brand products to buy and easy recipes to make, I feel confident that I can provide my family good nutrition without complaints! I'm not a dietician and I need someone to just plain tell me how much is good and bad!"

—Beth R., mother of two

"As the mother of two boys always on the go with sports, scouts, etc., I am always looking for quick nutritious meals that I can feel good about. Janice and Liz have done it with creative, easy-to-make meals that use foods I typically have in my kitchen. I have selected many new recipes to try on my family."

—Susan L., mother of two

The Moms' Guide to Meal Makeovers

The Moms' Guide to
MEAL MAKEOVERS

Improving the Way Your Family Eats,
One Meal at a Time!

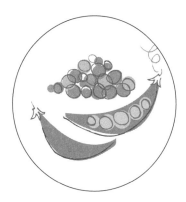

Janice Newell Bissex, M.S., R.D.,
& Liz Weiss, M.S., R.D.

BROADWAY BOOKS / NEW YORK

Broadway Books titles may be purchased for business or promotional use or for special sales. For information, please write to: Special Markets Department, Random House, Inc., 1745 Broadway, New York, NY 10019.

PRINTED IN THE UNITED STATES OF AMERICA

BROADWAY BOOKS and its logo, a letter B bisected on the diagonal, are trademarks of Random House, Inc.

Visit our website at www.broadwaybooks.com

First edition published 2004

Illustrated by Laura Coyle

Library of Congress Cataloging-in-Publication Data

Bissex, Janice Newell.
The moms' guide to meal makeovers : improving the way your family eats, one meal at a time! / Janice Newell Bissex and Liz Weiss.
p. cm.
1. Cookery, American.   2. Quick and easy cookery.
3. Nutrition.   I. Weiss, Liz.   II. Title.

TX715.B49945 2004
641.5'55—dc21
2003051925

ISBN 0-7679-1423-6

1 3 5 7 9 10 8 6 4 2

For Carolyn & Leah

— JANICE

For Josh & Simon

— LIZ

CONTENTS

ACKNOWLEDGMENTS

I t's one thing to say you want to write a book but it's another thing altogether to actually sit down and do it. There were many people who contributed to the successful completion of this book. First, we would like to thank our literary agent, Jenny Bent, for making *The Moms' Guide to Meal Makeovers* a reality. Her creative input, honesty, and wonderful sense of humor helped guide us through the long and often challenging process. Jenny, you're the best!

Writing a book with 120 recipes required a lot of time in the kitchen, mountains of dirty dishes (which Janice's husband, Don, usually washed), and friends and family willing to taste and test them. Those who had no choice in the matter included our husbands, Don Bissex and Tim Carruthers, and our children, Carolyn Bissex, Leah Bissex, Josh Carruthers, and Simon Carruthers. You were the best guinea pigs we could have ever asked for. Thanks for tasting our recipes, both the fabulous ones and the flops, and offering your feedback. We are also grateful for your patience during the many hours that it took to research and write this book.

It would be impossible to thank everyone by name who offered ideas, recipes, a cup of flour (whole wheat, of course), and encouragement throughout this long process, but please know that we appreciate your support. We would be remiss without acknowledging certain groups and individuals including Diane Newell, Pat Donovan, and Katherine Musgrave for reviewing and critiquing sections of our manuscript, and Lolly Tharp for assisting with some of our recipe development. Many thanks to photographer Joe Turner, who did a great job with the photo on the back cover, and to Grace Andrews and Joe Nardone for offering their kitchen as a beautiful backdrop. We also appreciate the offbeat humor and terrific work of Rich Brooks and his team at flyte new media on the development of our website, www.mealmakeovermoms.com.

Our sincere thanks go to the hardworking staff at Broadway Books, especially our editor, Patricia Medved, and her assistant, Beth Datlowe; publicist, Heather Maguire; director of publicity, Suzanne Herz; marketing manager, Julia Coblentz; and designer, Elizabeth Rendfleisch. We would also like to extend our utmost appreciation to Laura Coyle for her whimsical illustrations and cover design.

Janice would personally like to thank her friends and recipe testers at the Melrose Unitarian Universalist Church, especially Catherine Cezeaux and Maryellen Fitzgibbon. She is also indebted to her neighbor and good friend, Mary Hayward, for helping out whenever needed. Without the support and assistance of her parents, Dave and Carol Newell, Janice could never have embarked on such a huge project. She thanks them from the bottom of her heart. Janice also acknowledges the valuable contributions that her siblings Jeff, Lori, Denise, and Diane have made (especially the product research and recipe testing on the West Coast). Last, but not least, Janice thanks her husband, Don, for always going above and beyond and supporting everything she does.

Liz would like to acknowledge her neighbors, the Lopes, Richardson, and McGlinchey families, for tasting dozens of her recipes. Teenager Andy McGlinchey raved over our Simply Delicious Broccoli, confirming that it's possible to prepare veggies so that kids will not only eat them, but enjoy them. Liz thanks her parents, Bob and Sylvia Weiss, for the culinary and emotional support that she needed to complete the project, and her two sisters, Marian and Amy.

Finally, we'd like to thank each other for staying focused, sticking to deadlines, and working as a team. Finding humor in all the little (and big) bumps in the road kept us going strong and made the experience of writing this book well worth the effort.

INTRODUCTION

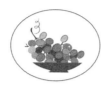

I t's 4 P.M. and if you're a mom, we'll bet that you—like a staggering 60 percent of all Americans— don't have a clue what you're having for dinner tonight. After all, you're busy. You work hard at home or at the office, and as much as you'd like to, you don't have a lot of time to think about dinner. The clock keeps ticking and soon pizza, macaroni & cheese, frozen fish sticks, chicken nuggets, or fast food becomes dinner tonight.

Sound like your house? Well, even though we're dietitians, we're also moms, and we have to admit that we've struggled with the same thing. In fact, the scenario we just described happens all over America—busy moms (who, by the way, still do most of the cooking) relying on take-out or frozen and boxed convenience meals to feed their families. The kids love it, there's no muss or fuss, but the drawback is that little twinge of guilt you feel every time you feed your family another marginally healthy meal. Remember, we're moms, too. We've been there. We feel your pain . . . and your guilt.

We know how hectic life as a mom can be and understand that although you really want your family to eat right and live a healthier life, making that happen can often be a challenge. So as fellow moms, we're here to help. Don't worry. We promise not to spend the next 300-plus pages outlining one of those rigid food plans that advocates eating things like lowfat, high-protein, or no-sugar foods all day. Diets like that don't make sense over the long haul and your family will look at you like you're nuts anyway. What we'll do instead is suggest a family meal makeover—a diet renovation, if you will—with plenty of realistic guidelines and easy-to-fix family recipes designed to bring super nutrition to your family's table.

If you think good nutrition takes too much time and effort . . . if a green vegetable has never passed your child's lips . . . or if you fear your family would rebel if you switched from white bread to whole wheat, then read on and discover just how easy and delicious a meal makeover can be.

Bear in mind that as you incorporate our strategies into your everyday life, you will automatically join the ranks of other Meal Makeover Moms (a drumroll, please) committed to improving the way their families eat. Your meal makeover journey need not begin and end with this book, however. By visiting our website, www.mealmakeovermoms.com, you'll have an opportunity to join the Meal Makeover Moms' Club. As a member, you can trade time-saving tips with other moms, share advice on surviving life in the mealtime trenches, customize your own grocery shopping list, and submit recipes for us to make over. Other benefits to joining the Meal Makeover Moms' Club include a monthly newsletter and new recipes for your family. We hope you'll join the club!

A Note from Janice:

In my house I have a 90/10 rule. That is, if we eat healthy 90 percent of the time, I don't worry too much about the other 10 percent. This leaves room for treats like cookies at Nana's house, an occasional fried seafood platter, and root beer floats on hot summer afternoons.

I admit that I secretly pray during dinner that my daughters will eat their vegetables because I know how important they are to good health. But if they've had a glass of orange juice at breakfast, half a banana or mango slices for a snack, and cantaloupe, grapes, or carrots with lunch, I don't stress if my children don't eat all their vegetables at dinner one night. Not making a big issue over what my girls do or do not eat is something I work on, since trying to convince (or bribe) kids to eat certain foods is usually counterproductive in the long run. All we can do is offer a variety of delicious and nutritious foods: What and how much they eat is up to them.

I wrote this book because I know the challenges and frustrations of trying to feed finicky eaters. With all my knowledge about food and nutrition, even I have gone through a "short-order cook" phase of preparing macaroni & cheese several nights in a row when it was the only thing my kids would happily eat. Of course I used a healthy brand with no artificial ingredients (Annie's Homegrown), made it with olive oil and lowfat milk, and then served it with berries or melon slices on the side!

As a mom and a dietitian I've learned a lot over the years about feeding kids. Now, with *The Moms' Guide to Meal Makeovers,* I'm glad to be sharing my insights with you.

A Note from Liz:

When I was growing up, the kids next door had this awesome candy closet that they were allowed to raid any time of the day. Boy, was I jealous. As much as I begged my mom for that same endless supply of licorice, gumdrops, and lollipops, she never caved in. While in my house we often had a small sweet treat after dinner, my neighbor's carte blanche policy on candy sure seemed a lot more appealing at the time.

Well, now as I reflect on that infamous candy closet, I can see the wisdom in my mother's household rules. The last thing she wanted us to do was to fill up on sugary sweets when she was busy making delicious, colorful, and hearty dinners for us most nights.

Like mother, like daughter. Today, as a mother of two hungry boys, ages seven and four, my own food philosophy reflects my mother's. I truly enjoy making healthy and appealing meals for my family. Trust me, when I cook, it's usually quick and easy, but that doesn't mean I'm willing to compromise on good nutrition.

One of my goals with *The Moms' Guide to Meal Makeovers* is to help you feel comfortable establishing your own family's mealtime rules and, even more important, to show you how to stick to them. With the advice and recipes presented in this book, your job of providing nourishing meals for your family (yes, often day in and day out) will become manageable, fun, and ultimately a simple way of life.

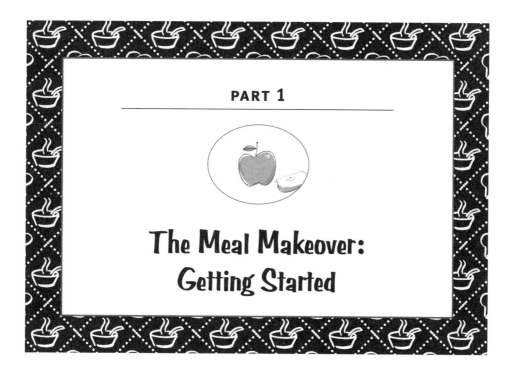

PART 1

The Meal Makeover: Getting Started

It's a jungle out there. Supermarkets tempt us with buy-one-get-one-free promotions on sugary and salty junk foods but rarely on healthy stuff like broccoli and bananas. Fast food companies entice our children with free toys and special meals that, unbeknownst to many moms, can contain nearly 1,000 calories and over 40 grams of fat. And television ads target our children with offers of prizes, even cash, for buying sugary breakfast cereals and candy. It's easy to see why lots of people get coaxed into eating too much and too many of the wrong kinds of foods. Indeed, it can be frustrating. But instead of blaming everyone else for the deterioration of the American diet, we think it's time for moms to take control of the situation. The good news is that you don't need a degree in nutrition or advertising to improve the way your family eats. All you need is an experienced guide to show you the way. That's where we come in: the Meal Makeover Moms.

Part 1 of our book is our rallying cry to bring moms like you to the front lines of change. After all, if moms don't take a stand against all the forces that sabotage good nutrition, then who will? We are confident that after you read Part 1, eating well will become second nature. Here's what we mean: Say, for example, you're making tuna sandwiches for lunch. Rather than the usual tuna and mayo on white bread, you can simply add a shredded carrot to the mix and use whole wheat bread instead of the usual white. With little effort, your meals get a quick makeover with the addition of fiber and health-enhancing nutrients from the whole wheat bread and the carrot.

Our goal is for you to learn how to seize good nutrition opportunities at every turn . . . from stocking a healthy pantry to getting your kids to try new foods without the usual fuss at the table. Here's what's in store as you read on:

• **Chapter 1:** *Why Do Families Need a Meal Makeover?* In this chapter, we'll tell you what's wrong with today's "all-American" diet and explain why a record number of adults, children, and teens are now overweight or obese. But rather than dwell on the negative, we'll outline our Super Simple Nutrition Guidelines, a framework for eating well and adding extra nutrition to everything you and your family eat.

• **Chapter 2:** *The 5-Step Meal Makeover Plan* If your family is currently eating a C-minus diet, this chapter will take them to a B-plus . . . or even better. Our plan is practical and realistic with tips for jump-starting your family's meal makeover, marketing good nutrition to kids (if junk food companies can do it, so can you), establishing food rules no respectable Meal Makeover Mom should be without, streamlining your time in the kitchen, and eating together as a family.

• **Chapter 3:** *The Best of the Bunch* When and if you serve your family convenience meals such as frozen chicken nuggets, boxed macaroni & cheese, and frozen pizza, we'll reveal which products and brands are the best tasting and most nourishing ones out there. We'll also offer Quick Fix Tips for weaving extra nutrition into those meals. And if your family eats fast food, we'll give you strategies for cutting back on your visits and decreasing the amount of calories, unhealthy fats, and sodium you consume when you do find yourself at the drive-thru.

• **Chapter 4:** *The Meal Makeover Pantry* In this chapter, we'll show you how to stock your pantry with everyday, wholesome ingredients—things like canned beans, salsa, frozen greens, nuts, and whole wheat pasta—that make last-minute cooking healthier and easier. With a well-stocked pantry, you won't have to rely as much on take-out, fast food, and the pizza delivery man.

With the information and tips in Part 1, you'll be well on your way to a healthy meal makeover. So roll up your sleeves and get started.

CHAPTER 1

Why Do Families Need a Meal Makeover?

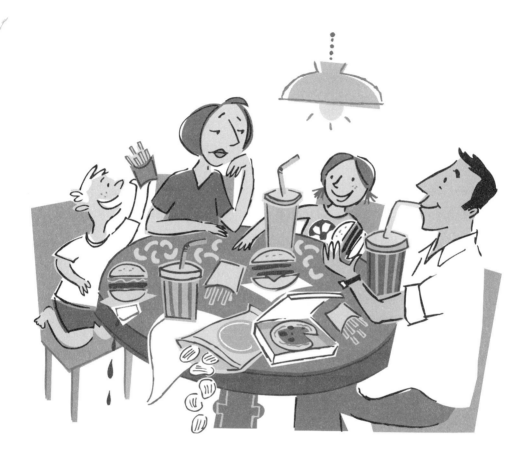

We'd like to begin this chapter on a positive note, so we'll start by saying: "You're amazing." You run in a million different directions all day—working, carpooling, volunteering, buying birthday presents, folding laundry, picking up toys, making beds, flushing toilets (let's not get too graphic here), setting up play dates, and hopefully squeezing in a quick workout. But just when you want to sit down and catch your breath, IT'S DINNERTIME! You scramble to pull something, just anything, together because everyone is hungry and homework still needs to get done. Somehow you do it. You manage to feed your family. Maybe it's not the same homemade meal your mom cooked when you were a kid (you know, the one with the meat, starch, and vegetable every night). But yes, it's behind you. Later that evening as you fold the last load of laundry, your day as a supermom is coming to a close. Yeah . . . you made it!

It's tough to do it all and do it all well. In fact, for years now, we've been talking to busy moms like you who say they're often too dog-tired to cook meals or pack school lunches and therefore way too tempted by all the convenience foods designed to make life easier. There's no doubt that the foods we've come to rely on—hot dogs, chicken nuggets, frozen pizzas, mac & cheese, lunch kits, take-out, soft drinks, snack chips, and fast food—have meant less time in the kitchen. It's hard to imagine life without them. But unfortunately all that convenience has come at a nutritional price.

Today, Americans eat 340 more calories per day than they did just two short decades ago. Sugar consumption is at an all-time high, and the number of refined carbohydrates that we eat—white bread, bagels, hamburger buns, muffins, crackers, pastries, white rice, and pasta—dwarfs healthier, high-fiber whole grains. And even though fruits and vegetables are readily available in supermarkets, most families don't make a habit of eating them at every meal. To add insult to injury, Americans are less active today, thanks in part to modern conveniences like cars, elevators, and drive-thru windows as well as leisure activities that revolve around the TV or computer. It's no wonder a growing number of children, teens, and adults are now considered overweight or obese. But besides our nation's battle with the bulge, many people—overweight, skinny, or anywhere in between—are opting for nutritionally stripped-down foods that provide little in the way of vitamins, minerals, phytonutrients (plant nutrients), and fiber—the very things that fight heart disease and cancer, protect our eyesight as we age, keep our skin looking young, and so on and so on.

Today's families can benefit greatly from a meal makeover. For your family, that makeover may end

Statistics to Chew On

- Sixty-one percent of U.S. adults are overweight or obese.
- Thirteen percent of children (ages 6 to 11) and 14 percent of teens (ages 12 to 19) are overweight.
- Children are more active than their parents, though 42 percent of girls and 26 percent of boys do not exercise vigorously on a regular basis.
- In 1991, 42 percent of U.S. children were enrolled in daily school-based physical education classes. The number dropped to just 29 percent in 1995.

up being a simple one . . . like switching from blue eye shadow to a more flattering brown (oh, what were we thinking back in the eighties?). For others, it may be more extreme. Either way, the changes you bring to your table (large or small) will provide a lifetime of benefits, including feeling better, looking better, and staying healthier.

There's Trouble at the Table

FOOD: WE EAT TOO MUCH

Last summer, Liz and her husband took sons Josh and Simon to an amusement park. It was one of those hot, you-could-fry-an-egg-on-the-sidewalk sort of days, so they all decided to cool off with an ice cream cone. The trouble with the cones that Liz ordered, however, was their size: They were colossal. What Liz had asked for were four "kiddie" cones, but what she got were cones so large that even the adults could barely finish them.

Whether you're eating at a restaurant, fast food establishment, or even at home, standard portion sizes of everyday foods have gotten bigger and bigger. In a recent study comparing common portion sizes in 1977 to those consumed nearly twenty years later in 1996, researchers actually proved that Americans are indeed eating a lot more food than they used to.

Portion Sizes on the Rise: Changes Observed from 1977 to 1996

FOOD ITEM	INCREASE IN PORTION SIZE	INCREASE IN CALORIES
Salty Snacks	0.6 ounce	93 calories
Soft Drinks	6.8 ounces	49 calories
Fruit Drinks	3.8 ounces	50 calories
Hamburgers	1.3 ounces	97 calories
French Fries	0.5 ounce	68 calories
Mexican Dishes	1.7 ounces	133 calories

Source: *JAMA*, January 22/29, 2003-Vol 289, no. 4.

In the United States, there has been a definite trend toward "supersizing," now considered a significant factor in our growing rate of obesity. Consider that a person who adds just 100 extra calories to his or her diet each day without then burning those calories off will gain 1 to 2 pounds of body weight per year. Over a ten-year period, that's 10 to 20 more pounds on the waistline! Standard por-

Portion Pointers

Heaping 5 cups of pasta into one dinner bowl does not a portion make. In fact, the USDA considers just ½ cup of cooked pasta to be a "portion." To keep portion sizes in check—so you don't end up eating 10 pasta servings in one sitting when 2 servings is more realistic—check out the portion size recommendations listed below.

BREAD, CEREAL, RICE, AND PASTA

1 slice of bread

½ cup cooked cereal, rice, or pasta

1 ounce ready-to-eat cereal

1 tortilla

3 to 4 crackers

FRUIT

1 whole fruit (medium apple, orange, banana)

½ cup chopped, cooked, or canned fruit

¾ cup fruit juice

½ grapefruit

¼ cup dried fruit

VEGETABLES

1 cup raw leafy vegetables

½ cup cooked or canned vegetables

7 to 8 carrot sticks

1 medium potato

¾ cup vegetable juice

(Source: USDA)

MILK, YOGURT, AND CHEESE

1 cup milk

8 ounces plain or flavored yogurt

1½ ounces natural cheese

MEAT, POULTRY, FISH, DRY BEANS, EGGS, AND NUTS

2 to 3 ounces cooked lean meat, poultry, fish

1 egg

2 tablespoons peanut butter

½ cup cooked beans, peas, lentils

⅓ cup nuts

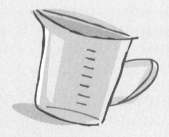

tions have increased slowly over the years, right before our very eyes. The change has been so gradual that our brains and stomachs have simply increased their capacity for bigger platefuls of food.

SUGAR: WE EAT TOO MUCH

It has been said that Americans are conspicuous consumers of sugar. In fact, on average, people eat about 33 teaspoons a day (that's a whopping 528 calories from sugar alone). How much is too much? Well, consider that a person who consumes 2,000 calories a day is advised by the USDA to limit his or her intake to just 10 teaspoons or 40 grams of added sugar a day. To put that number in perspective and understand how quickly sugar can add up, consider that 1 cup of Frosted Flakes has 4 teaspoons (the same as four Oreo cookies), a 12-ounce soft drink contains 10 teaspoons, one Dunkin' Donuts coffee cake muffin has nearly 15 teaspoons, and a medium fast food chocolate shake contains about 20 teaspoons of added sugar. Sugar by itself isn't a villain, but keep in mind that sugar-laden foods often provide a lot of calories, few nutrients, and tend to displace more nutritious foods in the diet, including fruits and whole grains.

More than 20 percent of the added sugar in the U.S. food supply comes from one source: soft drinks. According to the National Soft Drink Association, the "average" American consumes 57 gallons of soft drinks a year (the equivalent of 20 ounces a day). Sugars are everywhere. They're in cookies, cakes, donuts, syrups, and sugary breakfast cereals. Some unlikely foods may also contain added sugar, namely hot dogs, pizza, soup, lunchmeat, fruit drinks and sports drinks (perhaps a bit more obvious), flavored yogurt, salad dressing, and some peanut butters.

REFINED GRAINS: WE EAT TOO MANY

Sugary foods aren't the only Achilles' heel of the American diet. As a nation, we're also hooked on fluff . . . and we don't mean the sticky, sweet white stuff in a jar. By fluff, we mean all the white, refined flour used for making bagels, muffins, hamburger buns, pizza crust, white bread, crackers, tortillas, cookies, and pasta. We eat more flour today than ever before. And therein lies the problem. We simply eat too much of it. In fact, on average, Americans consume about 10 servings of grain-based foods a day. And of those 10 servings, just 1 is a fiber-rich *whole* grain (experts advise eating at least 3 whole grains a day). So instead of choosing things like whole wheat bread, brown rice, whole grain breakfast cereals, whole wheat pasta, and whole wheat couscous, we're grabbing for fluff . . . and missing out on all those good things found in whole grains: fiber, zinc, vitamin E, and other phytonutrients.

Eating whole grains offers protection against heart disease and certain cancers. They're also filling—a bonus for folks watching their weight—and promote healthy digestion (something you can appreciate if you or someone in your family suffers from constipation, the number one gastrointestinal complaint in the United States). Whole grains offer a big bang for the nutritional buck.

Snack Attack

Kids love to snack. A recent survey of school-age children found that 80 percent do it once or twice a day. Snacks account for 20 percent of a child's daily calories, but sadly, some of the most popular snacktime choices are those with the least nutritional value. Soft drinks rank number one while fruit weighs in a distant twelfth. But parents can take advantage of their children's snack attacks by offering healthier nibbles like fruit, nuts, lowfat yogurt, popcorn, or vegetables with dip.

What Kids Are Snacking On:

1. Soft drinks
2. Salty snacks such as potato chips, corn chips, and popcorn
3. Cookies
4. Non-chocolate candy
5. Artificially flavored fruit beverages
6. Whole milk and chocolate milk
7. 2% reduced-fat milk
8. White bread
9. Chocolate candy
10. Cake
11. Ice cream
12. Fruit

(Source: National Health and Nutrition Examination Survey III)

FATS: WE EAT THE WRONG KINDS

Okay. We're about to make a confession that may surprise you but here goes . . . *we love fat.* Yes folks, you heard us right. We love to cook our food in a tablespoon or two of olive oil or canola oil. We enjoy snacking on a handful of nuts. We're crazy about guacamole. We can't imagine a plateful of steamed broccoli without a flavorful drizzling of extra virgin olive oil on top. We could sing the praises of fat all day long. Bear in mind, however, that nowhere in our confession did we say we love lard, the skin on chicken, or the hydrogenated oil and shortening found in crackers, cookies, and many other processed foods.

Fiber Fallout

Fiber isn't technically a nutrient because our bodies can't digest or absorb it. But fiber contains a bundle of health benefits. It lowers heart disease risk, promotes healthy digestion, and may even play a role in the prevention of colon cancer. Fiber is found only in plant foods . . . things like fruits, vegetables, whole grains, and beans. In fact, it's the fiber that gives plants their structure. In other words, without fiber, asparagus, carrots, celery, and green beans would resemble limp spaghetti. It's not surprising that most kids don't make the grade when it comes to eating enough fiber. Just how much fiber do kids need? New federal guidelines suggest that children between 1 and 3 years old need 19 grams of fiber per day, kids 4 to 8 need 25 grams, and older kids need between 25 and 38 grams per day, as do most adults. A 3-year-old would meet his fiber requirements by eating two slices of 100% whole wheat bread, ½ cup broccoli, a small banana, ¾ cup Cheerios, a handful of raisins, and a serving of our Last-Minute Black Bean Soup.

Although rumors abound that fat makes you fat and raises blood cholesterol levels, the honest truth is that not all fats are created equal. To set the record straight, fat won't make you fat . . . eating too many calories without burning them off will put on the pounds. Also, while saturated fat and trans fats can raise your blood cholesterol level, monounsaturated and polyunsaturated fats will do just the opposite. Once you discover the difference between the good, the bad, and the ugly, we hope you and your family will learn to appreciate the health and culinary benefits of fats and oils as much as we do (and without guilt, we might add).

The Good Fat

• Monounsaturated Fats: While some folks are content to munch on fat-free cookies and crackers, we'd rather nibble on crisp apple slices slathered with all-natural peanut butter or French bread dipped in extra virgin olive oil. Eating foods rich in monounsaturated fats—olives and olive oil, canola oil, sesame oil, peanut oil, most nuts, avocados, and peanut butter—has been shown to reduce heart disease risk by lowering the so-called "bad" LDL cholesterol and increasing the "good" HDL cholesterol. People who live in Spain, Greece, Italy, and other Mediterranean countries enjoy diets rich in monounsaturated fats, and they also enjoy less heart disease!

• Polyunsaturated Fats: There are two types of polyunsaturated fats in the diet, omega-3 and omega-6. The vast majority of Americans get more than their fair share of omega-6 fats, found in things like corn oil and vegetable oil. Like the mono fats, omega-6 fats can also help to lower LDL cholesterol. The second kind of polyunsaturated fat, omega-3, is also good for cholesterol, but the benefits go well beyond heart health. Omega-3s are considered nutritional superstars, but unfortunately, most people don't eat anywhere near enough of them. They are found in fatty fish like salmon and trout in the form of DHA and EPA, the most potent form of omega-3. They're also present as alpha-linolenic acid in flaxseed (and products made with flaxseed such as breakfast cereals and waffles), walnuts, tofu, canola oil and canola mayonnaise, omega-3 eggs, unhydrogenated soybean oil, even Brussels sprouts and spinach. We think everyone should shift their fat focus to more omega-3s. Here's why: Omega-3s . . .

- Protect against heart disease by lowering blood pressure, making blood less likely to clot, and by improving blood lipid levels.
- Reduce the risk of sudden cardiac death by keeping the heartbeat stable.
- Are needed for brain and eye development in the fetus and young children.
- May help to treat autoimmune conditions including rheumatoid arthritis, psoriasis, and lupus.
- May play a role in the prevention and treatment of ADHD and other behavioral problems.

Interestingly, countries with the highest consumption of omega-3-rich seafood have the lowest rates of depression in the world.

The Bad Fat

- Saturated Fats: A big juicy steak, a mountain of mashed potatoes smothered in sour cream and gravy, and a few green beans swimming in butter may be the ultimate stick-to-your-ribs dinner, but it can also be the ultimate saboteur of your heart. Saturated fat, found in fatty meats, full-fat dairy products, lard, and tropical oils, gets a bad rap and rightly so: Eating too much of it can raise a person's bad LDL cholesterol and thus heart disease risk. Currently, about 13 percent of our total calories come from saturated fat, though experts recommend an intake of under 10 percent (that's about 20 grams a day for someone consuming 2,000 calories a day).

The Ugly Fat

- Trans Fats: What do vegetable shortening, stick margarine, and many microwave popcorn, fast food French fries, commercial baked goods, and even some lowfat cookies have in common? The answer is trans fats, created when vegetable oil is processed into partially hydrogenated vegetable oil. About 40 percent of the foods at the supermarket contain hydrogenated oils. Food companies use it to turn liquid oils into stick margarine and shortening and to extend the shelf life of everything from cookies to crackers. Trans fats are perhaps the ugliest of all the fats because they increase the bad LDL cholesterol while lowering the good HDL cholesterol. Currently, Americans get 2 to 4 percent of their daily calories from trans fats. It's a good idea, however, to eat as little as possible . . . a tall order since currently, it's tough to spot their amount in food products (food companies will be required to list trans fats on food labels by January 2006). Your best bet right now is to look for products that don't contain hydrogenated oils or shortening.

SALT: WE EAT TOO MUCH

Americans eat between 3,500 and 4,000 milligrams of sodium a day . . . far above the recommended 2,400 milligrams. Given the fact that you can consume well over 2,000 milligrams in one fast food meal alone, it's easy to see why some people have a hard time sticking to the guideline. Diets high in sodium have been linked to increases in blood pressure, so it's wise not to go overboard. While only 1 percent of children have high blood pressure, parents should still keep an eye on sodium. That's because children whose palates become accustomed to salty foods may be more likely to eat higher sodium diets as adults.

About 70 percent of the sodium in the typical American diet comes from processed foods like salty snack chips, canned soups, and convenience meals. Surprisingly, only 15 percent is actually added at the table or in home cooking. So if you're trying to limit your family's sodium intake, banning salt entirely from your cooking may have a smaller impact than you'd think. Instead of dwelling on the little bit of salt you may use in your recipes or at your table (and let's face it, adding salt to home-cooked meals can really help to kick up the flavor), focus instead on reading labels and choosing all those convenience foods wisely.

You can also try some of these other salt-slashing strategies:

• Drain and rinse canned vegetables and beans to wash away 30 to 40 percent of the sodium.

• Look for jarred pasta sauce with the least amount of sodium. Some have nearly 1,000 milligrams of sodium in just ½ cup while others contain less than 400 milligrams (see The Meal Makeover Pantry, Chapter 4).

• Switch to Diamond Crystal Kosher Salt for cooking and at the table. One teaspoon has 1,120 milligrams of sodium while 1 teaspoon of regular table salt has 2,325 milligrams.

FRUITS AND VEGETABLES: WE DON'T EAT ENOUGH

According to the USDA, the most frequently requested "vegetable" at the American table is French fries. That's pretty frightening! First of all, as Meal Makeover Moms we can't see the logic in calling a

Which Spuds for You?

SPUD STATS	1 MEDIUM BAKED POTATO	ONE 1.25 OUNCE BAG POTATO CHIPS	1 LARGE ORDER FAST FOOD FRENCH FRIES (160 GRAMS)
Total Calories	160	188	500
Total Fat (grams)	0.2	13	25
Saturated Fat (grams)	0	4	7
Trans Fats (grams)	0	variable	6
Sodium (milligrams)	17	225	888

French fry a vegetable. Sure, potatoes contain potassium, fiber, and vitamin C, but when you toss 'em into the deep-fat fryer and douse them with salt, the calories, artery-clogging fats, and sodium can quickly add up. In addition, when family members fill up on greasy French fries in lieu of fruits and vegetables, they miss out on all the amazing flavors that fruits and vegetables have to offer . . . not to mention all the health-enhancing nutrients.

So, for the record, let's just say that French fries aren't a vegetable. But once you take those fatty fries out of the mix and begin to analyze just how many fruits and vegetables people are really eating these days, research shows that most people eat nowhere near the recommended minimum of 5 servings of fruits and vegetables a day. It depends on whose data you look at, but we've seen figures that show just 20 percent of Americans meet the goal. Young children between the ages of 2 and 12 fare even worse with only 4 percent eating enough fruits and veggies each day.

When you think about how and where families eat these days, it's easy to see why the 5-a-Day goal is so challenging. For starters, Americans eat one in every three meals away from home. In addition, on average, 10 percent of a child's daily calories come from fast food (and how many kids do you know who order a salad when they're at McDonald's)? Other barriers to eating more produce include the fact that busy home cooks tend to use fewer ingredients when making dinner and prepare fewer vegetable and grain-based side dishes than their mothers did years ago.

PHYSICAL ACTIVITY: WE DON'T GET ENOUGH

One of the biggest reasons Americans are just about the plumpest people on the planet is the fact that few get the recommended 30 minutes or more of moderately vigorous exercise each day. Hey, we know it's tough. We're die-hard New Englanders and, trust us, it's not much fun walking to the bus stop when it's 10 degrees outside. But we bundle up and "just do it." The benefits of regular physical activity include:

- Weight control
- Strong bones and muscles
- Better self-image
- Lower risk for diabetes, heart disease, and some cancers

Sure, we could tell you to take the stairs versus the elevator, kick a soccer ball around with your kids, and encourage you to turn your kids on to sports and physical activity over surfing the web . . . but you already know that. What we thought we would do instead is show you how even a small amount of movement can make a huge impact on your family's health.

Consider this: If your child got off the couch and did just one of the following activities every day, he would burn an average of 26,500 extra calories each year. For an overweight child, that small increase in activity alone could lead to a $7\frac{1}{2}$-pound weight loss.

Calories Burned (based on an 80-pound child)	
20 minutes of running around the playground	50 calories
20 minutes of crazy dancing in the family room	55 calories
15 minutes of brisk walking	65 calories
30 minutes of bike riding	75 calories
20 minutes of playing soccer	120 calories

Calcium: Do Your Kids Get Enough?

Children today are in a calcium crisis. Only 13 percent of teenage girls and 32 percent of teen boys get the recommended daily amount. Diets low in calcium put kids at risk for osteoporosis—the brittle-bone disease—later in life.

During childhood, bones grow rapidly and reach their peak bone mass by around the age of twenty. That's why it's critical for children and teens to do everything they can to build the strongest bones possible, while they have the chance. To do that, it's important to get regular exercise and to eat a diet rich in calcium. Children ages four to eight need 800 milligrams daily while those ages nine to eighteen need 1,300 milligrams. Milk, at 300 milligrams per cup, is one of the best calcium food sources but it's not the only source. Consider the following:

- One cup of lowfat fruited yogurt has 385 milligrams of calcium.
- Two calcium-fortified waffles or one glass of calcium-fortified orange juice has the same 300 milligrams of calcium as a glass of milk.
- One cup of cooked broccoli has 180 milligrams.
- One orange contains 52 milligrams of calcium.
- One glass of calcium-fortified soymilk also has 300 milligrams.
- Snacking on ¼ cup of almonds provides 80 milligrams.
- Fast food, despite its nutritional shortcomings, can be a quick source of calcium.

> 2 slices Domino's Vegi Pizza = 280 milligrams
>
> 1 Wendy's Broccoli & Cheese Baked Potato = 200 milligrams
>
> 1 McDonald's Fruit 'n Yogurt Parfait = 250 milligrams
>
> 1 McDonald's Cheeseburger = 250 milligrams
>
> 1 Wendy's Chocolate Pudding = 57 milligrams

FYI: Our bodies need other nutrients including vitamin D (the sunshine vitamin) for optimal calcium absorption. Some good vitamin D food sources include milk, fortified cereal, and eggs.

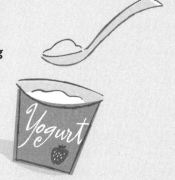

Just Tell Us What to Eat

The two of us have worked as registered dietitians for over twenty years now, and a request that we often hear from fellow moms is: "Just tell me what to feed my family." Our answer is a simple one: Get back to basics. Sure we could impress you with all the latest buzzwords on nutrition: ketosis, glycemic index, syndrome X, and the Zone. But you know what, all those fancy terms and fad diets are irrelevant and almost laughable when you're trudging through the supermarket with three kids in tow and they're all begging for Cocoa Puffs at the same time. Honestly, you have better things to do than stress over ketosis or the role of polyphenols in the diet. Hey, don't get us wrong. The science of nutrition is fascinating, but do you really have the time or the mental strength to sit there with your calculator analyzing how many grams of carbohydrate or protein your family just ate for dinner? It's not realistic, nor is it much fun.

Your meal makeover journey is about to begin with our Super Simple Nutrition Guidelines. Nothing we are about to tell you is rocket science, yet everything we are about to recommend is indeed based on science . . . good science. The best way to use our guidelines is to first take a closer look at your own family's diet. If iceberg lettuce and French fries, for instance, were the only two veggies at your table this week, then our first guideline, Enjoy a Rainbow of Colorful Fruits and Vegetables Every Day, may be something to start striving for. By being more mindful of the basic principles of healthful eating, the road to super nutrition is easier to follow.

MOMS' SUPER SIMPLE NUTRITION GUIDELINES

1. Enjoy a Rainbow of Colorful Fruits and Vegetables Every Day
- Eat at least 5 servings a day . . . even more is better.
- Choose from all the colors—blue/purple, green, yellow/orange, red, white—to benefit from the super nourishing nutrients in each color category.
- Eat fruits and vegetables "as is" or add them to casseroles, soups, stews, smoothies, desserts, and much, much more.
- Opt for locally grown or organic produce whenever possible.
- Eat fruits and vegetables fresh, frozen, or canned . . . it all counts!

2. Go with the Grain . . . the Whole Grain
- Make at least 3 of your daily grain servings whole grain.
- Prepare sandwiches with 100% whole wheat or whole grain breads, pitas, and wraps.

- Switch to breakfast cereals with at least 2 grams of fiber per serving.
- Go out of the box by cooking with more whole wheat pasta, bulgur, couscous, and brown rice.

3. Be Finicky about Fat

- Choose olive oil and canola oil as your main cooking oils.
- Make foods that contain omega-3 fats (salmon and other fatty fish, canned tuna, canola oil, walnuts, and foods made with flaxseed) a regular part of your family's diet.
- Lower saturated fat by choosing lean cuts of meat and reduced-fat dairy products, removing the skin from chicken, and curbing your fast food intake.
- Decrease trans fat consumption by limiting foods made with hydrogenated or partially hydrogenated vegetable oil or shortening.

4. Select Nourishing Beverages and Snacks

- Drink water throughout the day.
- Choose 100% fruit juice rather than sugary fruit "drinks." (Note: The American Academy of Pediatrics recommends limiting daily consumption of fruit juice to 4 to 6 ounces for one- to six-year olds and 8 to 12 ounces for seven- to eighteen-year olds.)
- Select calcium-rich beverages such as lowfat milk, soymilk fortified with calcium, and calcium-fortified orange juice.
- Eliminate or cut back on soft drink consumption. (Note: If your child drinks one soft drink a day, try weaning her to one per week. After one year alone, she'll drink 29 fewer gallons and shave 50,000 calories from her diet.)
- Offer more nourishing snacks, including fruit, yogurt, nuts, whole grain crackers, popcorn, lowfat cheese sticks, fruit smoothies, and baby carrots with dip.

5. Pick Good-for-You Protein Foods

- Eat more nonmeat protein foods, such as beans, nuts, and tofu (they're all naturally low in saturated fat).
- Strive for two fish meals a week.
- Don't be afraid of eggs, a high-quality protein food packed with important nutrients, and shop for omega-3 eggs whenever possible.
- Seek out the leanest cuts of beef and pork, reduced-fat luncheon meats, and lowfat dairy.

6. Balance Food Intake with Physical Activity

- Enjoy 30 minutes of physical activity most days of the week.
- Eat when hungry, stop when full.
- Keep a watchful eye on food and beverage portion sizes when eating at home, at restaurants, and at fast food establishments.

Okay. So now you're sitting there thinking, "Yeah right! Like my kids are ever going to eat this way." Trust us, they will. We can say that honestly because we're right there in the mealtime trenches with you and understand your challenges. So don't get worried. We're not going to tell you to feed your family more green vegetables without giving you strategies for how to actually do that successfully, nor will we suggest you go cold turkey on fast food without providing appetizing alternatives. What you need is hands-on advice . . . advice that works. So read on, because what's in store will change your family's eating habits forever.

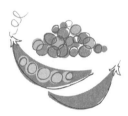

Most of us don't eat with a calculator by our side. However, to put the latest nutrition recommendations into perspective, we've offered a general guideline for what a person consuming 2,000 calories a day should eat.

- Limit total fat to 65 to 75 grams per day
- Limit saturated fat to less than 20 grams per day
- Limit sodium to less than 2,400 milligrams per day
- Eat about 250 grams of carbohydrate per day
- Eat 25 to 35 grams of fiber per day
- Consume 75 to 100 grams of protein per day

CHAPTER 2

The 5-Step Meal Makeover Plan

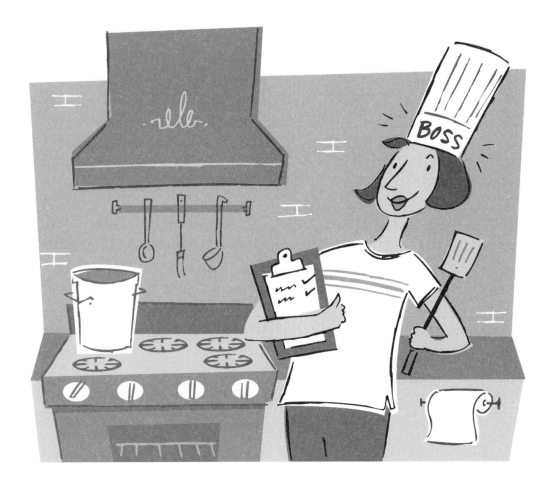

Now that you have a better sense for the kinds of nourishing foods your family should be choosing each day, one big question remains: What's the best way to actually get your family to eat this way? Rome wasn't built in a day, so don't expect your kids to give up the Twinkies and Fruit Roll Ups overnight. However, with our 5-Step Meal Makeover Plan, healthy eating habits can eventually become part of your everyday life. If this sounds too good to be true, it's not. As you'll soon learn, a family meal makeover involves more than offering an apple for an afternoon snack or carrot sticks in a lunchbox, though that is a great start. It's a new way of thinking about food.

Our 5-Step Meal Makeover Plan begins with the commitment to actually take those first tentative steps toward change. Make them small steps. That way, they'll help you gradually improve your family's eating habits over the long haul. Giant leaps, as you can only imagine, often end in frustration and failure, so don't go there. If your family is currently eating what might be considered a C-minus diet, this first step, *You Have to Start Somewhere,* can help to jump-start your journey to a B. Don't stress over trying to eat A-plus meals day in and day out because perfection is hard to come by and not always realistic (trust us, we know this from firsthand experience). *You Have to Start Somewhere* is your brand-new beginning.

Our second step is where you get to be fun and creative in the kitchen by marketing good nutrition to your family. Think about the millions of dollars fast food companies spend marketing burgers and fries to your kids with incentives like online kids' clubs and free toys. We'll give you a crash course in marketing and show you how to compete with the likes of fast food restaurants and soft drink companies. And don't fret, you won't have to pay your children money or give them gifts every time they eat a green vegetable. They'll eat it because it looks and tastes great.

Step 3, *Establish Food Rules,* gives moms the a-okay to get tough. Remember, you're the queen of the kitchen, and although we live in a democratic society, you still get to set the rules on the types of foods you serve your family each day. Children of all ages may complain when parents set limits, but we know from research that kids thrive psychologically when consistent and thoughtful parental guidelines are laid out in front of them. You're going to love our rules!

You're also going to love Step 4, *Streamline Your Time in the Kitchen,* because after you read it, you'll become a lean, mean cooking machine in no time. Getting in and out of the kitchen in minutes, not hours, is the name of the game when you want to prepare nutritious and delicious meals for your family. Sure, you could grab the frozen fish sticks and Tater Tots, but by following the tips and suggestions presented in our fourth step, making meals from scratch will be just as easy (well, almost). If you've ever wanted to cook with the efficiency of a five-star chef, now's your chance.

Our final step seems like an obvious one, *Eat Together as a Family,* but as children get older and lives get busier, fewer actually do that. The fallout for kids who don't eat regular family dinners is a diet with fewer fruits and vegetables and more fried foods and processed convenience meals. To make matters worse, many families, while they may indeed eat their meals together, tune in to the television at the same time. This too can have a negative impact on a person's diet. We advocate eating as a family unit whenever possible . . . whatever your family unit happens to be.

Step 1: You Have to Start Somewhere

Have you ever run across one of those diet and nutrition books that tell you what you're *not* supposed to feed your family or make you feel guilty every time your child eats red meat, dairy, refined white flour, sugar, or salt? While the advice may be well-meaning, it's often downright ridiculous!

Let's get a few things straight. To be a Meal Makeover Mom, you will not have to recite the health benefits of niacin and zinc, nor will you be required to plant an organic vegetable garden in your backyard. Improving your family's diet doesn't have to be time-consuming or complicated. In fact, it can be a lot of fun. You just need a starting point.

NOT PERFECT, BUT BETTER

According to research from the USDA, most children between the ages of two and nine eat a diet that "needs improvement" or is "poor." In fact, only 36 percent of two- to three-year-olds and less than 20 percent of four- to nine-year-olds eat what the USDA would consider a "good" diet. It's easy to see why. At mealtime, children are more likely to eat French fries than any other vegetable, and most school-aged kids don't eat anywhere near the recommended minimum of 5 servings of fruits and vegetables a day. Today's youngsters consume half of their daily calories from fat and sugar, thanks in part to fast food and soft drinks. In fact, on average, children get 10 percent of their daily calories from fast food alone. Okay, you get the picture.

So where do moms begin? Well, for starters, we suggest you take small steps toward positive change. To do this, we advocate diet additions and trade-offs. Here's an example of an easy addition: Instead of banning frozen chicken nuggets from your household, you can still offer the nuggets, but now you'll be sure to also offer a vegetable or fruit on the side (see No-Nonsense Nuggets, page 276, and Moms' Best of the Bunch, page 54). For a healthy trade-off, swap the soda pop your family may be drinking with dinner with a fizzy mixture of 100% fruit juice and seltzer. If your family's diet is currently at "not so good," consider working your way to "not perfect, but better." Take it slow . . . one week at a time. Once you nail down one change, move on to the next. By the end, you'll have five new food habits to smile about.

FIVE WEEKS TO CHANGE

WEEK ONE: *Add One Extra Serving of Fruit Each Day*
• Most kids love cereal and will devour a big bowlful before heading off to school in the morning. This week, offer a serving of fruit *first*. When kids wake up and they're good and hungry, they'll gladly eat half a banana, some orange slices, or a small bowl of berries. One fruit serving down, and

then you can offer the cereal to complete the meal. If your children don't mind their food all mixed up, you can also toss a handful of berries or sliced bananas right on top of their cereal.

• As a change of pace from milk and cookies after school, make a naturally sweet fruit smoothie instead. In a blender, combine a cup of 100% fruit juice, ½ ripe banana, a handful of frozen strawberries (or any frozen fruit, for that matter), and ½ cup vanilla or fruited lowfat yogurt. Whip it up, pour into two or three separate glasses, and serve with a few whole grain crackers or graham crackers on the side.

• Children eat lunch at school about 180 days a year. If you pack their lunch or snack, add some fruit. Try grapes, sliced strawberries, cubed melon, a whole apple, or a single-serve fruit cup.

Week Two: Add One Extra Vegetable Serving Each Day

• If dinner is 5 minutes away, sit the family down and serve the evening's vegetable as an "appetizer." A few bites of broccoli, sweet potatoes, or crunchy raw vegetables with a salad dressing dip are all healthy ways to start the meal. Janice's three-year-old, Leah, happily sits in her booster seat nibbling on frozen peas or frozen corn while waiting for dinner. Even though they're still frozen, they're a lot of fun to eat.

• Hold the chips and Cheez Doodles and instead make baby carrots or grape tomatoes a regular side dish with your child's lunch.

• Drink your vegetables. In the juice aisle of your supermarket, check out some of the carrot and fruit juice beverage blends. One glass provides a day's worth of vitamins A and C. You can also use this juice for making your own freezer pops.

Week Three: Add One Healthy Beverage Each Day

• If you send your child to school with a sugary juice drink, switch to 100% fruit juice or 1% lowfat milk.

• A 12-ounce soft drink contains the equivalent of 10 teaspoons of sugar and about 150 calories. As an alternative, make your own fizzy creation of 100% fruit juice mixed with club soda or seltzer.

• Bring a plastic water bottle wherever you go for a quick thirst quencher. It will save you money and time when the kids say, "I'm thirsty."

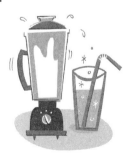

Week Four: Include One Healthy Snack Each Day

• For a nourishing midmorning snack, offer trail mix with dried fruit and nuts, a squeeze yogurt, or grapes. They're a delicious alternative to cookies and salty chips.

• If your cookie jar is filled with store-bought goodies—often made with unhealthy trans fats and a lot of sugar—make our easy Oatmeal Mini Chocolate Chip Cookies (page 326), Blueberry Snack Cake (page 330), or Our Favorite Chocolate Cookie (page 324) for a super-nutritious sweet alternative.

• Whenever you head out the door, whether it's to a soccer game or even to the supermarket, be sure to pack pretzels, dried fruit, popcorn, or an all-natural granola bar (read the label and go for the ones with the most fiber and the least sugar) in case the kids get hungry. Being prepared helps to avoid the inevitable visit to the vending machine.

WEEK FIVE: *Serve One Extra High-Fiber Grain Food Each Day*

• Reevaluate your breakfast cereals and switch from a sugary, low-fiber brand to one made with whole grains, containing 2 or more grams of fiber per serving. Some kid favorites that make the grade include Wheat Chex, Raisin Bran, oatmeal, and Cheerios. And remember, we're not striving for perfection here, so if your kids won't give up one of their sugary favorites, just mix it in with a healthier brand . . . you'll be 50 percent closer to your goal.

• Use 100% whole wheat bread and whole grain breads instead of white bread for sandwiches whenever possible. Many of the whole wheat varieties now available have a kid-pleasing soft texture.

• For a change of pace, use instant brown rice or whole wheat pasta instead of instant white rice or regular pasta. Check out our makeover recipes for Sweet & Nutty Thai Thing (page 178), Southwestern Chicken & Rice (page 292), Mini Meatballs with Whole Wheat Spaghetti (page 232), and more.

ARE FAT-FREE FOODS REALLY THE WAY TO GO?

Some experts will tell you that high-fat foods are unhealthy and that fat-free foods are the better way to go. In our opinions, nothing could be further from the truth. Some of the healthiest and most flavorful foods on the planet—nuts, olive oil, salmon, peanut butter, and avocados—are rich in health-enhancing monounsaturated and polyunsaturated fats, and we wouldn't give them up for the world. We firmly believe that if fat-free foods were *really* better for our overall health, then obesity and heart disease wouldn't be as rampant as they are today. Take fat-free cookies for example. Because they can lose some of their appeal when all the fat is removed, food manufacturers often replace the fat with more sugar. The result, ironically, is a cookie that contains about the same number of calories as the original. Since fat-free cookies are often perceived as healthier, people tend to eat more of them and hence consume more calories. Fat-free cheeses are another case in point where less is not necessarily better. We recently experimented with fat-free ricotta cheese for our Squishy Squash Lasagna (page 182). The fat-free version was lacking in flavor and had a somewhat grainy texture. In the end, we compromised and went for the reduced-fat ricotta. We managed to eliminate much of the saturated fat but kept the creaminess.

FAT ADDITIONS, SUBTRACTIONS, & TRADE-OFFS

BEFORE	AFTER	HEALTH BENEFIT
Whole milk	1% lowfat milk or skim milk	Less saturated fat and calories (Whole milk is recommended until the age of two.)
Full-fat cheese	Part-skim or reduced-fat cheese	Less saturated fat and calories
80% lean ground beef	93% or 95% lean ground beef or lean ground turkey	Less saturated fat and calories
1 sleeve fat-free cookies	2 regular full-fat cookies	Fewer calories, better taste (You can stop at 2.)
Reduced-fat peanut butter	100% all-natural peanut butter	More heart-healthy monounsaturated fats
Stick margarine and vegetable shortening	Tub, liquid, or trans-free margarine	Less trans fats
Butter	Olive oil and canola oil	More heart-healthy monounsaturated and polyunsaturated fats

While it's always our goal to cut unnecessary calories and as much artery-clogging saturated and trans fats as possible, we would never tell you to eliminate foods rich in mono- and polyunsaturated fats, the types that promote good health. Our chart above offers some simple substitutions that keep a moderate amount of monos and polys on your table while nixing much of the saturated and trans fats.

Ready, Set, Go!

When parents put pressure on themselves to provide perfectly healthy meals 365 days a year, they can burn out. Achieving perfection at the family dinner table is close to impossible, and it's certainly not realistic given today's busy lifestyles. We believe you'll have better success as a Meal Makeover Mom if you forget perfection and strive for small positive changes instead.

Go ahead and replace sugary breakfast cereal with a whole grain brand that helps to boost your child's nutrient and fiber intake. Rather than grabbing for that jumbo bag of chips, consider some crunchy nuts in its place. And by all means, offer an extra fruit serving every day. Adding a handful of healthy foods to your child's diet here and there, making wise trade-offs, and realizing that some days will be better than others are all simple ways to begin your family's meal makeover. Sure, it would be easy to toss in the towel, but if you simply make the commitment to start somewhere, you'll be able to relax, enjoy the ride, and begin your journey to change.

Step 2: Market Good Nutrition to Kids

Before we explain some of our savvy strategies for marketing good nutrition to children, consider the stiff competition. Every day, American children are bombarded with television advertisements for sugary cereals, candy, salty snacks, and fatty fast foods. During Saturday morning television, for example, nine out of ten food advertisements tout junk food over fruits, vegetables, and other healthy fare. When was the last time you saw a TV ad promoting broccoli? Given the fact that youngsters average 28 hours of television viewing a week and are exposed to over 20,000 advertisements a year, it's easy to see why some prefer Big Macs to big bowls of fruit salad.

Television advertisements are literally just the tip of the food marketing iceberg. Every time a food company places its logo on a child's toy, game, school supply, T-shirt, or baseball cap, it is effectively advertising and promoting its product. If your children surf the web—and currently, millions do—they are targeted with online advertisements for a host of products, including foods and beverages. Additionally, since many popular kid foods are strategically placed at the child's eye level in the supermarket, when your sons and daughters spot their favorite superhero on a box of breakfast cereal they probably do what many kids do: beg you to buy it.

Yogurt Wars: Liz Strikes Back

Liz can certainly relate to the superhero supermarket scenario. While the average supermarket stocks about 35,000 food items, Liz's two boys managed to home in on just *one* of those food products on a recent shopping trip. It all began when Liz and sons Josh, age seven, and Simon, age four, were walking down the dairy aisle. As they approached the yogurt section, the kids noticed something they had seen advertised on television. "Look, Mom," they cried. "Those are the new Star Wars yogurts with glow-in-the-dark lightsaber tubes. Can we get them, Mom? Please, please, please!" What the kids were referring to was the popular Go-Gurt portable snack yogurts . . . you know, the kind you can eat without a spoon. While for years Liz had been buying a different brand called YoSqueeze (don't you love these names?), the kids insisted on the new ones.

Let the Yogurt Wars begin. Liz's first reaction was to take a closer look at the label. Both the original brand that Liz had been buying and the one with the Star Wars packaging contained roughly the same amount of fat and calories. But as Liz read on, she noticed things like artificial color and flavor . . . something she tries to limit whenever possible (for the sheer fact that kids get plenty of the artificial stuff elsewhere). Was Liz going to give in to this savvy marketing gimmick or would she stick with the all-natural yogurt she and the boys had always loved? To avoid a full-blown battle, she was tempted to grab Darth Vader and run for the nearest escape pod. Instead, she stood her ground and offered the kids a crash course on the powerful influence of advertising. So the next time you're faced with a similar predicament, take the opportunity to teach your children how to be clever consumers. Follow our tips and "may The Force be with you."

• Explain to your children how advertisements are designed to make products look more exciting so people will want to buy them.

• Discuss how you can't judge a product by its packaging any more than you can judge a book by its cover. In other words, just because a superhero or superstar athlete is on a box of cereal doesn't mean it tastes good or is good for you.

• Conduct a blind taste test between the brand your children want and the one you prefer. Chances are, they'll agree that Mom's choice tastes just as good if not better. (Liz's seven-year-old took the yogurt taste test and declared Mom's choice as the winner.)

• Look at labels and point out how many of the most heavily advertised cereals and snack foods are often loaded with the most sugar, hydrogenated oil, artificial colors, and artificial flavors.

Moms' Marketing Tactics: Give Good Nutrition a New Spin

Given the choice between beets and French fries, which would your children prefer? Okay, so our question seems a bit silly. Beets aren't exactly the most appealing kid food on the planet. But what if we told you that with some clever Madison Avenue–style marketing, there's a chance your kids would choose (or at least try) the beets? You may think we're kidding, but we're really serious!

Robin, a mother of two, gets her girls to eat all sorts of colorful vegetables, including beets. How does she do it? First, she buys fresh beets, scrubs them, trims the ends, sprinkles them with olive oil, salt, and pepper, and then wraps them in foil. The beets are placed in a baking pan and roasted in a 400°F oven until they're tender. They take about an hour to cook and once the outer layer is peeled away, the end result is sweet, delicious, and incredibly beautiful beets that according to Mom are "to die for." The bottom line here is that it's possible to get your kids to eat just about anything as long as you make it appealing. That's what we mean by marketing.

Tempt the Senses

The biggest challenge with getting kids to try a new food is persuading them to take that very first bite. Even if the food is delicious, chances are your child won't open his mouth if it doesn't look good. Children and adults eat with their eyes. When we were creating the recipes for this book, Janice's ten-year-old daughter, Carolyn, served as our reality check, reminding us that if a dish was "ugly," as Carolyn used to put it, there was no way it should go in the book. As a result, what you will find are recipes that tempt the senses and thus encourage kids to try new things. Imagine a dinner table filled with Walnut-Crusted Salmon (page 258), Simply Delicious Broccoli (page 318), and Chocolate-Dipped Strawberries (page 335). With an array of colors and shapes, the meal becomes a marketable alternative to the bland-colored chicken nuggets and potato puffs that some children might be accustomed to eating.

Your next challenge is to make the food taste good. One way to do that is to lightly season your food with salt (we prefer the flavor and lower sodium content of Diamond Crystal kosher salt), herbs, and spices and to avoid the temptation to make your meals fat free. Fat gives food flavor and is a key component of a healthy meal makeover. The trick is to choose the right kinds of fats and to use them in moderation. For example, with the help of a small amount of olive oil and some garlic, we transform plain old spinach into mouthwatering Garlicky Sautéed Spinach (page 316). Even the occasional pat of butter melted on peas or green beans is okay, especially if it makes the vegetables more appealing. A tablespoon here or a teaspoon there can do wonders for the flavor of a meal and help you on your way to marketing good nutrition to your family.

Be a Good Role Model

If the old saying "do as I say, not as I do" applies to mealtime at your house, chances are your children will quickly catch on. If you grimace at the sight of peas or proclaim your objection to oatmeal every time it's served, you really can't expect your children to try, let alone eat them. And if you dash out the door in the morning without eating breakfast, getting your kids to eat their morning meal may be a tough sell as well. Since youngsters learn how to walk, talk, and eat a varied diet by imitating what they see, parents and caregivers can set a good example by making healthy food choices. Think of this as an opportunity to improve your own eating habits, too.

Research has confirmed that adult food choices play a key role in what children prefer. In one study, it was shown that young girls were more likely to drink milk versus soft drinks if their mothers drank milk themselves. So remember, whether you're serving beets *or* brownies, eat it with a smile.

Take the Medicine Out of the Meal

Do you ever find yourself saying things like "eat your carrots, they're good for your eyes" or "you'd better finish your milk so you get strong bones"? While we fully support teaching children about the health benefits of eating a well-balanced diet, all too often parents leave taste out of the conversation. Take vegetables, for example. By touting their healthy attributes and nothing more, children may come to believe that vegetables don't taste good. In the end, your kids might reject green beans and broccoli the same way they refuse their cough medicine. When you "have to" eat a certain food, it can take the pleasure away. The next time you're trying to encourage your children to eat their carrots and drink their milk, entice them by saying, "These carrots are delicious and sweet" and "This ice-cold milk is so refreshing, let me know when you want more." By taking the medicine out of the meal, some of the foods your children may have reluctantly forced down in the past can become foods they look forward to eating.

Try New Foods Over and Over and Over Again

If you're like us and find yourself running or driving your minivan in a million different directions, you probably have little time to plan or prepare dinner. Sure, it's tempting to take the easy road by offering the no muss, no fuss fast food and convenience meals that kids will surely eat. But in order to market good nutrition to children, it's important to expand their food horizons. The challenge, however, is that research shows it can take ten to twenty tastes over the course of many meals before a child eventually learns to like a new food. For Liz's son Simon it seemed more like forty tries before broccoli became his favorite vegetable. At some meals, he actually tasted the broccoli but most nights it landed on the floor or was flung across the kitchen. Liz persevered and always (well, almost always!) kept a level head. She never coerced or bribed young Simon to eat his broccoli, nor did she get angry or make a big deal when he rejected it umpteen times. Children love attention, whether it's positive or negative, so if they know you're getting frustrated at the table, they'll continue the behavior. Our advice, having been there, done that, is to hang in there. Just put the food out and avoid making a big issue about who ate what.

We can all learn a thing or two from the multibillion-dollar advertising industry that bombards us with so many advertisements that we're often persuaded to buy something new. The same can be said for repeating a child's exposure to a new food. The more often the food is offered, the better the odds that your child will taste it and add it to his or her list of favorite foods. And remember, there are dozens of fruits and vegetables to choose from, so if you fail with one, move on to the next (just don't forget to come back to those old "castoffs" later).

Offer the Three Cs: Choice, Creativity, and Compromise

Kids are control freaks. That's why it's critical to present them with plenty of choices throughout the day. Choices come in handy when you're trying to market good nutrition. For example, rather than tell your kids they "have to eat some fruit with dinner," consider a more positive approach by giving them a choice between two different fruits. "Do you want watermelon or grapes . . . or both?" Given the choice, they'll probably pick at least one. The same goes for vegetables. "Do you want zucchini or carrots tonight?" Trust us, it works most of the time.

It's also important to be creative. We don't mean you have to make smiley faces on pancakes (unless, of course, you enjoy doing that sort of thing). But experiment a bit with your usual array of recipes by trying some new ones that may be a little different from what the kids are used to. In other words, take a few small steps "out of the box" in order to pique their taste buds and curiosity about food. Our makeover recipes are designed to do just that (check out our Moroccan Un-Stuffed Peppers, page 284, and we're sure you will agree). With creativity you can also make up fun and silly names for foods. Telling your five-year-old that "this broc rocks" may get her to try broccoli. Hey, it's worth a try.

The last of the three Cs is compromise. It's unrealistic to expect any child—teen or toddler—to eat A-plus meals seven nights a week. Come to think of it, it's unrealistic to expect adults to eat this way either. There's room for compromise, and we believe it can actually help your efforts to market good nutrition. If, for instance, the kids have been begging for hot dogs all week, there's no reason to deny them. While we don't advocate hot dogs as everyday fare, one of our Best of the Bunch hot dogs (page 55) is certainly a fine choice once in a while. And if the children want chips on the side, don't feel guilty if you end up doling out a handful or two. To round out the hot dogs and chips, however, consider some crunchy baby carrots and sliced strawberries or mango as well. Everyone wins.

Cook Meals Together

If you're worried that cooking with the kids will be time consuming, messy, and chaotic, you're right. But it's a heck of a lot of fun and can spark lively conversations on family food traditions, where foods come from, and of course, good nutrition. When Janice peels carrots before dinner, three-year-old Leah "assists" while nibbling on a carrot of her own. Liz's boys love to help with their favorite Blueberry Banana Pancakes (page 152), munching on frozen blueberries along the way.

Sure, on the nights when you're strapped for time, it may be best to let the kids watch their favorite video for twenty or thirty minutes or send them outside to play. But when there's time, we suggest you invite your kids into the kitchen. Children who help with a meal are more willing to take a few bites and perhaps try something new. Helping hands make food more enjoyable and kids feel proud when they know they've been part of the process. Just keep your broom and sponge handy, because you'll need them.

Marketing Genius

Food companies spend billions of dollars advertising their products. That's power. But guess what: You've got the power, too. Now that you've learned some new marketing strategies, you may even get your kids to eat Brussels sprouts. All it takes is the following: Rather than expect your children to eat plain old boiled Brussels sprouts, now you can kick up the flavor 150 percent by steaming them until very soft and then tossing with butter, olive oil, garlic, pine nuts, kosher salt, and Parmesan cheese (see Finally Edible Brussels Sprouts, page 317). Brussels sprouts—which, by the way, are a rich source of bone-building vitamin K—can be delicious and appealing to kids. It's all a matter of how you make and market them. So the next time you find yourself pinned to the wall and worn down by repeated attempts to get your family to eat a varied diet, consider some of our savvy marketing strategies. You just may be surprised by your own success.

Step 3: Establish Food Rules

Imagine what life would be like without rules. As much as your child may gripe when you tell her to "clean your room," "look both ways before you cross the street," "do your homework," and "brush your teeth," children need structure. They need to know what's expected of them in order to develop both emotionally and socially. When it comes to food rules, however, many parents feel guilty when they have to impose limits and restrictions. One reason may be that children often whine, cry, and complain when they're told they can't have candy before dinner or soft drinks with meals. Sometimes it's just easier to cave in. However, in order to move ahead with your family's meal makeover, you'll need to lay down the law. Luckily, you don't have to be a dictator to do so.

To establish realistic rules, child development experts recommend making them specific, reasonable, and enforceable. For example, if you tell your children that soft drinks and candy are forbidden, chances are you won't be able to enforce it, since kids spend a lot of time outside of the home where you have no control over what they eat or drink. A more reasonable approach might be a rule stating that soft drinks are off limits at meal and snack times but allowed on special occasions such as birthday parties. While the food rules you institute may be different from ours, the following five rules can easily be adapted to every family, no matter how old the children may be.

RULE 1: MOM IS THE EXECUTIVE CHEF, NOT THE SHORT-ORDER COOK

The title of Executive Chef implies that you are "the boss" and that's exactly what we mean by this first rule. As Executive Chef, you get to set the menu and decide what's for dinner. Sometimes, busy moms run out of dinner ideas or get burned out from all the complaints. When that happens, they toss in the dish towel and, out of sheer desperation, morph back into a short-order cook. Hey, we've all been there.

To attain and maintain your status as Executive Chef, plan only one meal, but make sure it's delicious and nutritious with some familiar components so the kids are more likely to eat it. It's also a good idea to serve one or two dishes on the side (such as sliced fresh fruit, carrot sticks, or whole wheat bread), just in case your main dish isn't well accepted. That way there's something for everyone.

Another reason moms end up cooking on demand is that their children often refuse to take even one bite. That's a real dilemma because no one likes to force a child to eat something he clearly doesn't want to eat or to send him to bed hungry. To encourage your children to try new things, we suggest you serve "No Thank You Bites" of everything. Here's how it works: Say you've prepared our No-Nonsense Nuggets (page 276) for dinner along with Maple-Glazed Carrots (page 313) and a side of grapes. Everyone—including Mom, Dad, and the kids—is required to place at least one bite of each item on his or her plate. If one of the children, for example, doesn't want the nuggets, you still serve him a "No Thank You Bite." At that point, you suggest he take a bite and say either "no thank you" or "thank you, I'd like more, please." "No Thank You Bites" provide a low-key and often amusing way to introduce new foods and flavors to your family. Even if your child says "no thank you" a hundred times, one day he just may change his mind.

RULE 2: DROP OUT OF THE CLEAN PLATE CLUB

Young children have an innate ability to regulate their own food intake. In other words, they eat when they're hungry and stop when they're full. On some days, they might just pick at their meal while on others, they may devour everything and ask for seconds. If you're concerned that a scant forkful here or a spoonful there will result in starvation or malnutrition, you can breathe easy because over the course of a few days or a few weeks, your child will undoubtedly compensate by eating more. Some parents worry when their children pick at their food and some get frustrated by the waste. As a result, they establish "the clean plate club" to make sure no one leaves the table hungry and that nothing gets tossed in the trash. The problem with forcing a child to eat every last bite, however, is that it interferes with his or her own internal hunger cues. Telling a child he has to clean his plate before leaving the table or insisting he finish dinner in order to get dessert can result in overeating and may lead to obesity later in life. It can also make dinnertime a nightmare for everyone.

It's your job to present a variety of great tasting, nutritious foods, but it's your child's job to decide how much to consume at any given meal or snack. In the end, your children will learn to eat the calories they need. It's important to offer small child-size portions rather than the supersized portions we as adults have become accustomed to eating. A recent study found that when three-year-olds were served either a small, medium, or large portion of macaroni & cheese over the course of three days, they ate the same amount at each meal despite the increasing serving size. But when a group of five-year-olds was given those same three portions, they ate incrementally more food as the portion sizes got bigger . . . and apparently more tempting. The researchers concluded that somewhere between the ages of three and five, children actually learn to ignore their internal hunger signals and eat more when presented with larger portions.

As a rule of thumb, we suggest you serve your children small portions at the start of the meal. If they're really hungry, they'll clean their plates all on their own and then ask for seconds.

RULE 3: SERVE AT LEAST ONE FRUIT AND VEGETABLE AT MOST MEALS . . . AND IT DOESN'T HAVE TO BE GREEN

When planning meals, think variety. Even if it's one of those days when you're shuttling the kids from soccer practice to piano lessons and a box of macaroni & cheese is the only thing you can muster up for dinner, it's still possible to round out the meal with at least 1 serving of a fruit or a vegetable . . . or better yet, both. If you're used to rotating through the same few fruits and vegetables at mealtime, break out of the rut by trying some new items from the produce aisle. For example, with your last-minute mac & cheese meal, serve some sliced mango, kiwi, or orange on the side. Remember, 1 serving of produce is only $\frac{1}{2}$ cup . . . an amount you could hold in the palm of your hand. So you see, upping your family's intake of fruits and vegetables is easier than you might think.

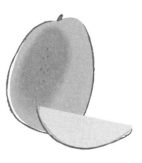

The Dreaded Green Stuff

As a parent, you have to be willing to lose a few battles, and getting your kids to eat spinach (or for that matter, any green leafy vegetable) may be one of them. A lot of moms believe green leafy vegetables are the be-all and end-all in the produce aisle. So when their kids refuse "the dreaded green stuff," they panic. While we advocate marketing green vegetables to children and adding them to recipes whenever possible, there's really no reason to stress when they're rejected, given all the appetizing and nourishing alternatives.

When we were growing up, our mothers told us to eat our spinach. After all, without it, how could we grow to be big and strong? We were so worried about being puny (and disobeying Mom!) that we forced down every last mouthful. Who wouldn't be ready for therapy after that ordeal? Well today, we're happy to report that our moms were wrong, sort of! The common belief back then, and even today, that spinach provides a hefty dose of iron in every bite is based more on the popular Popeye cartoon series than on popular science. It turns out that spinach does contain some iron, but it's in a form our bodies can't readily absorb.

So if spinach isn't the best source of iron, then why is it so highly regarded? Among other things, bright green vegetables, as well as ruby red strawberries, sun-kissed oranges, and sweet, mouthwatering mangoes, contain a host of plant pigments called carotenoids. Carotenoids act as powerful antioxidants in our bodies.

The Power of Antioxidants

You may have heard about antioxidants before but never quite understood why they are an essential part of a healthy diet. Antioxidants combat oxidation, a degenerative process that occurs naturally in our body cells as we age, especially when we're exposed to things like cigarette smoke, stress, and pollution. The result can be heart disease, cancer, and other age-related illnesses. A diet rich in a rainbow of colorful fruits and vegetables along with whole grains and things like nuts and seeds can help to keep oxidation at bay and literally keep us younger as we grow older. Since "the dreaded green stuff" is jam-packed with powerful antioxidants like beta-carotene, lutein, and zeaxanthin, we thought we'd tell you a bit about them and offer alternative ways to include them in your diet.

Beta-carotene is the best-known and most abundant antioxidant in the food supply.

It's found throughout the produce aisle in everything from spinach to squash. In our bodies, beta-carotene gets converted to vitamin A, a nutrient essential for normal growth and development, immune function, vision, and reproduction. Research shows beta-carotene may also ward off certain cancers and protect against heart disease.

Lutein and zeaxanthin are tough to pronounce (*lou-teen* and *zee-ah-zan-thin*) but both have been associated with a reduced risk for cataracts and age-related macular degeneration, the leading cause of blindness in the elderly. Foods rich in lutein and zeaxanthin include kale and spinach.

While green leafy vegetables are carotenoid superstars, other fruits and vegetables can also help to meet your daily quota.

BETA CAROTENE

WON'T EAT GREEN LEAFIES?	TRY THESE VEGGIES	TRY THESE FRUITS
Spinach	Broccoli	Apricots
Kale	Carrots	Cantaloupes
Turnip Greens	Sweet Potatoes	Mangoes
	Pumpkins	Peaches
	Squash	Nectarines
	Tomatoes	

LUTEIN AND/OR ZEAXANTHIN

WON'T EAT GREEN LEAFIES?	TRY THESE VEGGIES	TRY THESE FRUITS
Spinach	Yellow Corn	Red Grapes
Kale	Zucchini	Kiwi Fruit
Collard Greens	Peas	Persimmons
Romaine Lettuce	Orange Peppers	Pears
	Broccoli	Oranges
	Brussels Sprouts	Tangerines

RULE 4: LET THEM EAT CAKE . . . SOMETIMES

What kind of status does dessert hold in your house? Is it a reward for eating vegetables, strictly forbidden, or just one of the many delicious foods you offer your family? We believe the latter standing is the healthiest one for everyone.

When parents promise dessert in exchange for eating spinach, dessert becomes revered while the vegetable loses respect. In the end, children may perceive dessert as superior to the rest of the meal. On the other hand, banning dessert altogether may cause kids to want it even more. Cookies and cake taste great, so why forbid them? Our rule to "let them eat cake . . . sometimes" offers a happy medium, but it comes with a few caveats. While we believe that children should be exposed to a wide variety of great-tasting foods throughout the day, including sweet goodies, we're not talking carte blanche here. Our kids would eat sweet desserts all day long if given the chance, so instituting limits helps to ensure that children don't make saturated fat and sugar the mainstay of their diets. Given the fact that today's youth consume 50 percent of their total daily calories from fat and sugar, the *sometimes* part of this rule is especially important to enforce.

Many of the moms we've talked to over the years find it hard to believe that offering dessert can be one component of a healthy meal makeover. What we have found, however, is that by making dessert (i.e., one small cookie, a bowl of berries, one piece of chocolate candy) a part of the meal and not the grand finale, it becomes less of a big deal. But what if, for instance, on a particular night, one of your children only eats a few bites of dinner but demands dessert anyway? Our advice is to tell her to wait quietly at the table while everyone finishes their meal and that when dessert is eventually served, she's welcome to join in. In the end, while she's sitting there twiddling her thumbs, she'll probably realize she's still pretty hungry and may, in fact, eat more of her main meal.

Dessert Dos & Don'ts

• **DO** provide small dessert portions that satisfy a sweet tooth without going overboard on sugar, fat, and calories. A reasonable serving size for ice cream or frozen yogurt is ½ cup, not 3.

• **DO** break the mold by offering different types of desserts, such as fresh strawberries dipped in melted dark chocolate (see Chocolate-Dipped Strawberries, page 335), a juicy slice of watermelon, a frozen fruit juice pop, or Mandarin oranges topped with shredded coconut.

• **DO** sneak super nutrition into homemade desserts (see Deliciously Smart Desserts, Chapter 14).

• **DON'T** serve sweet goodies and other junk foods right before a meal, because chances are they will ruin your child's appetite.

RULE 5: PRACTICE GOOD MANNERS AT THE DINNER TABLE

While at first glance this rule may seem unrelated to good nutrition, without good table manners, mealtime can become chaotic and distracting. For example, if the kids are getting up and down from the table, burping on purpose just to get a laugh from a sibling, or sitting slumped in their chair, you may have little success introducing a new food or just getting the kids to eat their meal in general. When this happens, your children may still be hungry when they leave the dinner table, which can lead to hassles at bedtime when they want to raid the refrigerator for a big snack. When the kids forget their manners, parents lose control and the meal loses its appeal.

Everyone has different rules and philosophies about appropriate behavior at the table. Just remember, in order to enforce them, they'll need to be realistic. Consider some of our manner makeovers:

- **Stay in Your Seat.** Remind your children that once they leave the table, unless it's for a good reason such as getting seconds, dinner is officially over. Exceptions may need to be made for very young children.
- **Chew with Your Mouth Closed and No Talking with Food in Your Mouth.** No explanation needed here.
- **Use Inside Voices at the Table.** Screaming is not only annoying and disrespectful, it's also distracting . . . and distracted children don't eat well.
- **Say Please and Thank You.** Children who whine "Yuck, that meatloaf looks gross" can influence other siblings to also refuse the meal. A quiet "no thank you" or "yes, please" is a nicer way to communicate.

RULES ROCK

We believe that setting realistic food rules is one of the most important gifts you can give to your children. Food rules encourage healthy eating habits early in life, which ultimately lead to many benefits. The immediate advantages to your children are better health, a strong body, and more energy to learn and play. The long-term rewards are significant because they include lower risk of heart disease, cancer, osteoporosis, diabetes, and obesity, and a healthier relationship with food.

Step 4: Streamline Your Time in the Kitchen

A century ago, the average woman spent 44 hours a week preparing meals and cleaning up. Of course, convenience foods, take-out, refrigeration, and microwave ovens were nonexistent back then so getting dinner on the table was an all-day affair. Happily, things are a lot easier today, but like it or not, women still do the lion's share of the cooking. When the responsibility of preparing dinner seven nights a week, month after month, and year after year falls on your shoulders, it can become tedious and stressful to say the least . . . especially when it's 6 P.M., everyone is hungry, and the thought of starting dinner from scratch is nothing short of a bad dream. When time becomes a rare commodity, hot dogs, frozen pizzas, and fast food burgers become the inevitable dinner du jour. Clearly, time—or lack thereof—can be a big barrier to eating well.

For those of you out there who grew up at your mother's apron strings, you're probably more comfortable in the kitchen than those who grew up with Shake 'n Bake and TV dinners. But whether you're an old pro or are cooking family meals for the very first time, the key to kitchen happiness is efficiency. The tips and strategies outlined in Step 4 of our Meal Makeover Plan—*Streamline Your Time in the Kitchen*—are designed to turn cooking from a cumbersome chore into a more manageable commitment to your family's health.

USE CONVENIENCE FOODS BUT CHOOSE WISELY

Convenience foods can be the ultimate time savers. But if you're not careful, they can also be the ultimate diet saboteurs. The choice is yours, and trust us, the choices are many. Take some of those seemingly innocent packets of taco seasoning mix out there. Toss that packet into your favorite taco recipe and you can get 3,360 milligrams of sodium along with monosodium glutamate (MSG) and hydrogenated soybean oil. Even the 40%-less-sodium taco seasoning provides 1 teaspoon of salt per packet. While seasoning mixes may be convenient, they're not really a necessity when you consider that plain old chili powder, garlic powder, and cumin can provide the same Mexican-inspired flavors for less money and no added sodium. The bottom line on convenience foods: Read labels and choose wisely. While some items can get you in and out of the kitchen without compromising good nutrition, others are high in sodium, saturated fat, and trans fats (look out for hydrogenated oils listed on the label) and might be better off left on the grocery store shelf.

To save you time deciding which convenience foods to buy and which to forgo, you can read The Meal Makeover Pantry chapter, where we list our favorite convenience ingredients—everything from frozen broccoli florets to jarred pasta sauce—and offer brand-name recommendations as well as nutrition guidelines. You can also check out our chapter, *The Best of the Bunch,* where we evaluate frozen pocket sandwiches, frozen fish sticks, chicken nuggets, boxed mac & cheese, hot dogs, and other convenience meals . . . offering our "picks" for the best tasting and most nutritious brands in each category.

Kid Convenience

These days, it seems like entire supermarket aisles are devoted to children's snack foods. With loads of single-serve, individually wrapped options to choose from (peanut butter crackers, Gummie Bears, granola bars, and mini cookies to name just a few), they're the ultimate in convenience. But unfortunately, many contain gobs of sugar as well as unhealthy fats, including trans fats. Since trans fats are found in so many foods, it would be difficult to eliminate them entirely. The most realistic approach is to read the ingredients listed on food labels and limit your consumption of foods containing hydrogenated or partially hydrogenated vegetable oil or shortening whenever possible. Following are some of our favorite healthy snack options:

Makeover Moms' Grab-&-Go Snack Favorites

• **Fresh Fruit:** It comes in its own wrapper, requires little or no preparation, and is naturally packed with vitamins, minerals, phytonutrients (plant nutrients), and fiber.

• **Mini Applesauce:** Look for an all-natural brand and avoid the ones with added sugar and the fake blue, green, red, or pink coloring. What's up with that?

• **Mini Fruit Cups and Bowls:** Fruit cups and bowls come in handy when your own fresh fruit bowl is empty. Read labels and choose products packed in fruit juice versus syrup.

• **Squeeze Yogurt:** Go for the all-natural brands made without artificial colors and flavors.

• **Popcorn:** Our kids love the small bags of Smart Food and Boston Lite popcorn and we love the fact that popcorn is a whole grain. Look for popcorn made without hydrogenated vegetable oils. Popcorn isn't recommended until the age of four because it's a potential choking hazard.

• **Cheese Sticks:** Part-skim mozzarella cheese sticks provide high-quality protein and calcium and only 1 gram of unhealthy saturated fat.

• **Pretzels:** Choose whole grain or sunflower seed pretzels if they're available in your supermarket.

• **Granola Bars**: Look for granola bars made with healthy canola oil versus hydrogenated vegetable oils. Compare labels and choose the brand with the least amount of sugar and the most fiber.

• **Carrots with Dip:** Little packets of baby carrots with a ranch dressing dip are fun for kids and help to squeeze a vegetable into the lunchbox. A less expensive option is to pack a small bag of baby carrots with some dip on the side in a small plastic container.

• **Make-Your-Own Trail Mix:** Combine mixed nuts, raisins or dried apricots, mini pretzels, sunflower seeds, breakfast cereal such as Chex, and a few chocolate chips into a resealable plastic bag.

• **Crackers:** Read food labels and look for graham crackers and whole grain crackers made without hydrogenated vegetable oils.

The School Lunch Challenge

Okay. It's 7 A.M. and you're stuffing backpacks, braiding hair, pouring cereal, locating homework, and making school lunches. It's so hectic that it's easy to see why some busy moms grab for those ultra-convenient premade lunches. Hey, we won't call the nutrition police the next time you buy one, but remember that those easy-to-pack lunch kits (aka Lunchables) barely make the grade when compared to your own homemade lunch. When you read the following chart, you'll notice that our Moms' Lunch contains the same number of calories as the lunch kit. But our calories come packed with super nutrition: more protein, fiber, calcium, vitamin A, and vitamin C, and less saturated fat and sodium.

NUTRITION SCOREBOARD	LUNCHABLES "CRACKER STACKERS": LEAN TURKEY BREAST, AMERICAN PASTEURIZED PROCESSED CHEESE FOOD, AND RITZ CRACKERS. ONE REESE'S PEANUT BUTTER CUP, CAPRI SUN.	MOMS' LUNCH: OVEN-ROASTED DELI TURKEY AND REDUCED-FAT CHEESE ON WHOLE WHEAT BREAD WITH LIGHT CANOLA MAYONNAISE. BABY CARROTS, TANGERINE, TWO HERSHEY'S KISSES, 1% LOWFAT MILK.
Total Calories	430	425
Total Fat (grams)	19	12
Saturated Fat (grams)	9	5
Sodium (milligrams)	1,290	780
Total Carbohydrate (grams)	52	60
Fiber (grams)	1	7
Protein (grams)	15	24
Calcium	20%	45%
Vitamin C	0%	60%
Vitamin A	6%	180%

Run Your Kitchen Like a Chef

Is your pantry neat and tidy or in complete shambles? If you had to find a can of black beans or a jar of salsa right now, could you? How often have you found yourself in the midst of preparing a recipe only to realize—halfway through, of course—that you don't have a critical ingredient? While you dash to the store or to the neighbor's house to borrow it, dinner burns. And what about your shopping list? Do you even have one? If a professional restaurant ran its kitchen in the same disheveled manner as a lot of busy home cooks do, it would quickly go out of business.

For a restaurant to be successful, it's got to be well organized. We propose you adopt the same sort of efficiency. The good news is it won't cost you anything with the exception of some time (an investment that will save you wasted time in the long run).

Feng Shui Your Kitchen

Neither one of us knows much about feng shui (the ancient Chinese art of rearranging your living and working environment to improve every aspect of your life), but we've borrowed the term to stress the importance of getting your kitchen into shipshape condition. Carve out a few minutes now and then to organize your pantry. Knowing what's in your kitchen cabinets, refrigerator, and freezer and knowing exactly where everything is located can save you 5 or more minutes of search time every time you cook a recipe. Nothing could be more exasperating or more of a barrier to cooking fast meals for your family than rummaging through your kitchen every time you need a basic ingredient.

Something else to consider is the placement of your cooking equipment, tools, and ingredients. If you're cooking a meal at the stove but end up running to the other end of the kitchen to fetch your spatula, you're wasting valuable time. Do what restaurants do and keep all your kitchen essentials within grabbing distance. With an afternoon project devoted to rearranging your drawers and cabinets, you'll be well on your way to streamlining your time in the kitchen.

Shop Smart

Restaurants have the luxury of getting their groceries delivered to the back door every day. You, on the other hand (unless you grocery shop online), have to trudge to the supermarket regularly. It's not so bad unless you forget to add milk and eggs to your grocery list or shop without a list entirely. There's nothing worse than having to go back to the supermarket the next day for an overlooked ingredient.

What we propose is a customized shopping list, organized aisle by aisle. To help you create a personalized list, we've included a template on our web site, www.mealmakeovermoms.com. You can visit the site and tailor the list to your family's eating style. All you have to do is plug in the specific items you typically shop for into each column. Print out the list, keep it by your fridge, and when you're out of canned beans or frozen peas, for example, you can immediately check it off . . . before you forget about it. Refer to Chapter 4, The Meal Makeover Pantry, for a sample of our Makeover Moms' Shopping List.

Plan Your Menu

A lot of cookbooks suggest you plan your entire week's menu in advance. In theory, it's a great idea. Knowing what you're having for dinner seven nights a week helps to avoid that all-too-common 4 P.M. question: "What should I make for dinner?" However, planning ahead is not always realistic. And let's face it; while some people are genetically predisposed to being organized, others fly by the seat of their pants. But whether you're a "sit down on Sunday night and plot out the following week's menu" kind of person or you prefer walking in the door and whipping up a last-minute meal, both cooking styles can work to your advantage. All you need are two things: a well-maintained pantry and easy, nutritious, and family-pleasing recipes (see Part 2, The Meal Makeover Recipes).

Take our Last-Minute Black Bean Soup (page 106) as an example. If you have canned black beans, corn kernels, salsa, and preshredded reduced-fat Cheddar cheese on hand, you can create this hearty soup in under 15 minutes any night of the week . . . even if it's 6 P.M. and you just walked in the door. While knowing on Monday that you'll be making that dish on a Tuesday may take some stress off your shoulders, it's certainly a last-minute option as well. Follow our pantry guidelines and stick with our recipes and your meals will rival those of any restaurant.

Cook Like a Chef

Janice still laughs when she thinks back to the time her daughter insisted on making our chocolate pudding recipe all by herself. Carolyn, age ten at the time, refused Janice's help. Instead, she jumped right into the recipe, headfirst, neglecting to read it carefully or measure her ingredients ahead of time. Carolyn was doing fine for a while, whisking the pudding continuously, as the recipe instructed. Unfortunately, when it came time to add the yogurt and vanilla, she had to leave the stove, run to the fridge, find her missing ingredients, measure them out, and then add them. Lucky for Carolyn, the recipe worked out, but had she not located her ingredients right away, the recipe could have been a complete flop.

Who has not had a similar cooking experience? We certainly have.

To prevent a culinary faux pas such as Carolyn's, we suggest you cook like a restaurant chef and adopt a technique called *mise en place.*

Mise en place (meez-ahn-plahs) is a French term meaning "to put in place." Don't let the fancy French terminology intimidate you. This time-saving technique requires the chef or home cook to have every ingredient, utensil, and piece of equipment prepared and ready to go before the cooking begins. In other words, if a dish calls for a shredded carrot, a chopped onion, $1/2$ cup grated Parmesan cheese, and a lightly oiled baking pan, then all should be organized first. Using little bowls or cups comes in handy for holding ingredients until you're ready to cook. Of course there are always exceptions to this rule. If, for example, you're making a pasta dish for dinner, you can mise en place your ingredients while the water is coming to a boil or while the pasta is cooking. Mise en place makes cooking less hectic and more enjoyable.

Time-saving Kitchen Tools

Wouldn't it be great to win the lottery and spend some of the winnings on a new state-of-the-art kitchen? If we won, we'd install granite countertops, hardwood floors, not one but two high-end ovens, an island, a walk-in pantry stocked with every kitchen appliance known to mankind . . . you get the picture. Our dream kitchen would be designed with efficiency in mind. But you don't need an expensive kitchen makeover to get dinner on the table quickly. In fact, for less than $200, you can stock your kitchen with shortcut tools and be just as speedy. Here are a dozen items no Meal Makeover Mom should be without:

A Wet Paper Towel

Placing a wet paper towel under a cutting board stops it from sliding all over the counter as you slice and dice. A stable cutting board gets the job done quicker and it's also a lot safer.

A Sharp Chef's Knife

Dull knives just don't cut it when you're in a hurry. Besides the fact that they're more dangerous—you're more likely to cut yourself using a dull knife than a sharp knife—it takes a lot longer to slice, dice, and chop. You can buy a decent-quality chef's knife at any kitchen supply store starting at about $30. It's a great investment.

Kitchen Shears

Trimming the fat from chicken and meat can be difficult, even with the sharpest of knives. We rely on kitchen shears (aka scissors) to get this job done. They also come in handy when you're snipping herbs from your vegetable garden, cutting tortillas in half, and cutting bags of frozen vegetables open (it's a lot less messy than ripping them open and having half the contents fly out onto the kitchen floor). Most shears can be cleaned conveniently in the dishwasher.

A Good-Quality Vegetable Peeler

The old wives' tale that peeling carrots removes most of the nutrients is just that . . . a wives' tale. The outer skin on many vegetables is actually quite bitter, not to mention dirty, so peeling can often improve the flavor of your food. A good-quality peeler—versus that old hand-me-down from 1953—peels produce in a flash and costs less than $5.

A Box Grater

This four-sided grater has different-sized holes on each panel and is easier to handle and less messy to use than the one-sided washboard type. It's ideal for shredding a carrot (it takes less than 1 minute) and grating fresh ginger root.

Two Plastic Cutting Boards

To prevent cross-contamination (the spread of bacteria from one food to another), use one cutting board for raw meats, poultry, and seafood only and a second cutting board for ready-to-eat foods such as fruits, vegetables, and breads. We prefer a flexible cutting board for our ready-to-eat foods because it's easy to lift the board and transfer the contents—diced bell peppers, bread cubes, broccoli florets—into whatever we're cooking. Another benefit to two cutting boards . . . you don't have to waste time washing them between uses. Whether you use a plastic cutting board or a wooden one is a personal preference. We prefer a plastic cutting board because it is easy to clean and you can even run it through the dishwasher.

A Nonstick Skillet

A nonstick skillet (aka fry pan) allows you to cook with a lot less fat. By no means do we advocate fat-free cooking, but it's nice to know you don't have to use $\frac{1}{2}$ cup of oil every time you sauté something. Nonstick skillets make cleanup a breeze. We use a 12-inch skillet for everything from browning ground beef for tacos to cooking pancakes. A smaller 8- to 10-inch skillet comes in handy for cooking omelets or single grilled cheese sandwiches. You should be able to find a good-quality large nonstick skillet for about $30.

Adjustable Vegetable Steamer

Say goodbye to mushy vegetables. For under $10 you can buy a steamer and use it for cooking your family's favorite vegetables quickly and easily.

A Mini Food Processor

A mini food processor is a great time saver when chopping nuts or crushing corn flakes. If you do a lot of cooking, a full-size food processor may be worth the investment. A simple food chopper is also an option for chopping nuts, onions, garlic, and other veggies.

Blender

It's hard to make a fruit smoothie or to puree our Cheesy Broccoli Soup (page 116) or Orange Soup (page 112) without a blender. Expect to pay a minimum of about $30.

Whisks

Whisks come in many sizes and can do more than beat eggs. We use ours for mixing dry ingredients together instead of sifting and for incorporating flour into milk for thickening sauces.

Instant-Read Meat Thermometer

How many times have you wondered if your pork roast or chicken was thoroughly cooked? Take the guesswork out of cooking meat with an inexpensive (about $10) instant-read thermometer. This tool helps to avoid over- and undercooking.

LESS TIME, MORE NUTRITIOUS

It's a fact that women, even when they work outside the home, do more of the cooking than their husbands or partners. On average, women spend 45 minutes a day on food preparation while men contribute 13. When couples marry or move in together, women add an additional 4 hours a week to their housework load while men subtract about 3 hours from theirs. It's not our intent to depress you (although these statistics are a bit discouraging), but rather to get you thinking about clever ways to make over the way you prepare your family's meals. With time-saving strategies, you can streamline your time in the kitchen and create nourishing meals from scratch that take as little time as waiting for the pizza delivery man or heating up a frozen entrée.

Step 5: Eat Together as a Family

Which of the following scenarios best describes the dinner hour at your house?

Scenario One: It's 6 P.M., the table is set, your ten-year-old son is dutifully preparing a colorful salad and your toddler is playing quietly by herself. Minutes later, Mom, Dad, and the two smiling siblings sit down for dinner. A candle is lit and the mood is serene. Everyone eats the entire meal (including the vegetables) without complaint as they talk happily about their day. No one answers the phone when it rings. When dinner is over, the kids are excused, but not before clearing the table. Mom sits down to relax with the paper while Father and Son wash and dry the dishes.

Scenario Two: It's 5 P.M. and your toddler is so hungry and tired that he's having a major meltdown on the kitchen floor. Your teenage daughter is at soccer practice and your significant other won't be home until 7:30 P.M. You feed your toddler a quick meal of macaroni & cheese before whisking him off for his bubble bath and a bedtime story. Just then, your daughter barrels in from practice. You instruct her to change her clothes, wash up, and eat the leftover pasta that's still sitting on the stove. After she eats, it's time for homework. Finally, by 9 P.M., you and your partner sit down to last night's leftovers . . . but you're too exhausted to really enjoy them.

It's difficult to say just how many families actually eat dinner together on a regular basis. But it's clear from studies, surveys, and the latest statistics that the family dinner hour isn't what it used to be. For some families, coming together for dinner is a rare occurrence, while for others, it's still alive and well, albeit more challenging to coordinate. If you're finding it difficult to carve out time for family meals, we certainly understand. After all, more and more parents work outside the home nowadays and many children now participate in an array of extracurricular activities—sports, music, dance, karate, chess club, and drama—that often interfere with dinner.

We know it's tough, but eating together as a family is a key component of a healthy meal makeover. Studies have shown that sharing meals improves the family diet, strengthens family ties, enhances communication, fosters family traditions, and boosts self-esteem. Therefore, we hope you'll organize everyone's busy and divergent schedules to include regular family dinners. In other words, make it a priority.

FAMILY MEALS IMPROVE THE FAMILY DIET

We're happy to report that when families break bread together on a regular basis, they eat a healthier diet. Researchers at Harvard University confirmed this when they looked at the link between the frequency of family dinners and the quality of the diet among older children and adolescents ages nine to fourteen. They found that children who eat dinner with their families consume more fruits and vegetables and have a higher intake of fiber, calcium, iron, folate, and vitamins C, B6, B12, and E. Other conclusions:

• Eating family dinners is associated with a lower intake of fried food, soft drinks, saturated fat, and trans fats.

• Children who eat family dinners consume fewer frozen dinners, microwave meals, and other convenience entrées.

Turn Off the Tube During Dinner

Nixing TV during the family dinner hour (or half hour, or 20 minutes) may come as a shock to some family members. So to make your job easier, try some of our TV substitutions:

Movie Night: Establish one or two nights a month as "Family Movie Night." Rent a movie and let everyone watch as they eat.

Music to Your Ears: Every night, assign one family member the task of picking the background music for the meal.

Talk More: Replace the nightly drone of the TV with the buzz of your own conversation. At a loss for words? Buy a book designed to spark conversation such as *The Kids' Book of Questions*.

Tape It: If a favorite television show comes on during dinner, tape it on your VCR (hopefully you know how to program it) and then watch the program at a more appropriate time.

• Less than half of older children and adolescents eat with their families on a daily basis, with the frequency declining as children get older.

There are several reasons why eating dinner as a family improves the quality of a child's diet. For starters, Mom's (and Dad's) home cooking is typically a lot more healthful than the stuff older children might otherwise grab if left to their own devices—things like TV dinners, microwave meals, hot dogs, or popcorn. In addition, parents are a source of nutrition information, and the dinner hour offers a valuable time for teaching. And finally, when children eat meals outside of the home, they're less likely to eat fruits, vegetables, and whole grains.

TV TALK

We would be remiss if we neglected to mention the all-too-common practice of watching television during dinner. TV dinners—and we're not talking frozen food here—can undermine your family meal makeover in no time flat. Take a study from a few years back where the diets of children from families where the TV was normally on during two or more meals per day were compared to those of children from families with little to no mealtime viewing. The researchers found that the kids who tuned in to the tube ate more pizza, salty snacks, soft drinks, and meat, and fewer fruits and vegeta-

TV Trouble

While eating meals glued to the tube is a bad habit, watching too much TV in general can be a recipe for bad health. Research shows that obesity is highest among children who watch 4 or more hours of television a day and lowest among those who watch 1 hour or less daily. Remember, inactivity—a contributing factor to obesity—is fueled, in part, by television viewing. Other noteworthy statistics:

- The American Academy of Pediatrics recommends no more than 1 to 2 hours of TV viewing a day for children and no TV viewing until the age of two (a challenging goal to be sure).
- On average, children watch over 3 hours of television per day.
- Watching TV is the number one after-school activity for six- to seventeen-year-olds.
- Children spend about 900 hours in the classroom each year compared to 1,500 hours in front of the television.
- By age seventy, most people will have spent 10 years watching TV.
- The average child sees 20,000 TV commercials each year.
- Nine out of ten food ads on Saturday morning television are for sugary cereals, candy, salty snacks, fatty fast foods, and other junk food.
- Some studies have shown that when children watch TV, their metabolic rate (the rate at which they burn calories) is even lower than when they hang around doing nothing.

bles. What's more, the high-TV-viewing children also consumed twice as much caffeine as the youngsters with less screen time.

You don't have to be a scientist to appreciate the fact that when kids watch television, they zone out. One can only speculate that getting a five-year-old to try spinach for the very first time would be next to impossible with Batman blaring in the background. It's also clear that kids (and adults) whose focus is on their favorite TV show and *not* on their meal tend to eat mindlessly, and thus overeat. Another problem with television is the deluge of advertisements aimed at kids. Whether your children watch TV during the dinner hour or during other times of the day, commercial television bombards them with food ads, often touting sugary cereals, snacks, and soft drinks. These ads directly influence children's food preferences and can lead to tantrums at the supermarket when kids beg unmercifully for something they saw on TV.

FAMILY MEALS . . . MORE FREQUENT, MORE FUN

Okay. Hopefully by now we've persuaded you to eat together as a family more often. Just be realistic and remember: Every step toward change counts. If, for example, your family eats together once a week, perhaps bumping it up to twice or three times a week is a reasonable goal for you.

If you're too busy for family meals, perhaps you're too busy overall. Maybe it's time to cut back on one or two activities or to shuffle schedules around a bit in order to free up some time around dinner. By no means are we telling you how to run your life. It's just that we're so convinced about the benefits of eating together that it's hard not to be a strong advocate. To create a tradition of regular family meals in your home—even if your family is far from "traditional"—try the following strategies:

M.I.A.

It's not uncommon for at least one family member to be missing during the dinner hour. Perhaps Mom or Dad is working late that night and won't be home until 8 P.M., or a teenage son or daughter has basketball practice. Eating dinner at 8 P.M. is not always possible or desirable, especially with young kids, so instead, have everyone who is home eat together at the usual time. Save dessert, and when the missing family member comes home, reconvene around the table and eat together.

Be Flexible

If Dad consistently misses dinner because he's working late, perhaps he can come home 30 minutes earlier than usual once or twice a week *and* on those days, the family can eat 30 minutes later. Meeting halfway is a creative compromise and everyone wins. If this is impossible, then make time on the weekends, perhaps for Sunday brunch, when hopefully everyone is around.

Go Out of the Box

There's no rule that states a family meal has to take place at the kitchen table. Sometimes it's just not realistic. There are different ways and places to come together. For instance, if one of your children has a baseball game at 6 P.M., bring a blanket and a picnic dinner so everyone can eat together before or after the game. Going out for pizza (topped with vegetables, of course) on a Friday night when Mom or Dad is too tired to cook can provide a welcome break as well.

Plan Meals Ahead of Time

If 5 P.M. is meltdown time at your house, cooking dinner is the last thing you may want to be doing. To ease your stress, prepare meals or part of your mise en place ahead of time . . . perhaps the night before or during a young child's naptime. That way, things will be more tranquil when you sit down for dinner.

Make It a Habit

They always say habits are hard to break so make family meals a habit and you'll stick with them for a lifetime. The best time to start is when children are young and the family schedule is less demanding.

In addition to increasing the frequency of your family meals, remember to keep them positive and fun. The nightly ritual of breaking bread can strengthen family ties, but lecturing kids endlessly about table manners or berating them for their bad behavior earlier that day can cause a disconnect between family members. If dinner turns into a time to criticize and reprimand, the kids may dread coming to the table. Our advice is to make mealtime as enjoyable as possible so that everyone makes it a priority. To keep things upbeat and positive, try instituting the following table-time traditions:

Divide and Conquer

Preparing dinner night after night is one thing, but if you end up having to cook the meal, set the table, clear the dishes, load the dishwasher, and clean up, dinner can turn into a big drag. In fact, a recent survey reveals that the number-one challenge for moms at mealtime is getting the family involved in cleanup. Clearly, laying the entire burden of dinner on Mom's shoulders can be a major impediment to cooking nourishing meals. To lessen your load, we suggest you delegate. Consider assigning small mealtime jobs to every member of the family. One easy way to do this is to list all the chores, write them on separate pieces of paper, put them into a soup pot, and let the kids pick their nightly task. If your children are young, do what Janice does with three-year-old Leah and appoint a simple chore like laying napkins at everyone's place at the table.

Job List
- Set the table
- Prepare the salad
- Serve the meal
- Be the "runner" (the person assigned to jump up in the middle of dinner when someone needs more milk, etc.)
- Clear the table
- Load the dishwasher

Happy Talk

Asking your children "What was the best part of your day?" sounds a whole lot better than "I hear you were mean to your sister today." Ask positive, open-ended questions to ignite conversation instead of tempers. And remember to keep away from the running and often irritating commentary of who is eating what and how much since that can lead to tension at the dinner table.

Family Theme Nights

Establishing regular family theme nights such as "build-your-own-pizza night," "Mexican fiesta night," "banana split night," or "spaghetti & meatballs night" adds excitement to the meal and encourages children to try new foods.

Red Plate Special

When something exciting happens to a member of your family, such as a birthday, a good grade on a test, or a first homerun in T-ball, acknowledge the event with a special dinner plate. This distinctive plate can be red—as was used in early American times—or anything that will stand out at the table. It's a nice way of acknowledging someone's accomplishments.

Play Games

We're not suggesting you break out Monopoly at the kitchen table but consider other simpler games such as a Spelling Bee, GHOST, or the name game. At the Bissex house, a world map that hangs by the kitchen table sparks questions on geography and leads to all sorts of games, like "Where in the world is Ecuador?"

Set an Attractive Table

Bring the family's full attention to the table by lighting candles, using colorful napkins, or placing fresh flowers in the center.

Have a Dinner Date

Once a month, let each child invite a special friend for dinner. Your child can help you plan the menu and set a special table.

MEALS TO REMEMBER

When we were kids back in the sixties and seventies, our lives were less cluttered. There were no computers back then, nor was there instant messaging, after-school soccer games, karate lessons, or preplanned play dates. Our days were less complicated. Lifestyles have certainly changed over the past few decades, but for us, the importance of family meals has remained a constant. Indeed, gathering as a family after a hectic day evokes memories of a simpler time. Yes, we're nostalgic, but we're also realistic. We don't always live up to our mothers' example of home-cooked family dinners seven nights a week, but we try our hardest (and use plenty of shortcuts, we might add) because it's one tradition that makes a lot of sense for the well-being of our children.

If you are a Meal Makeover Mom striving to improve your family's diet, many of your efforts—from marketing good nutrition to establishing food rules—can come to fruition at the dinner table. Sure, some nights every elbow will be on the table and a recipe you've tried for the very first time may be a flop. But happily, you don't have to give up or get frustrated, because the next day or perhaps the day after when your family reconvenes for dinner, you can try again. Eating together is a ritual worth preserving. Your children will garner a lifetime of healthy food habits as well as delicious memories.

CHAPTER 3

The Best of the Bunch

Convenience & Fast Food

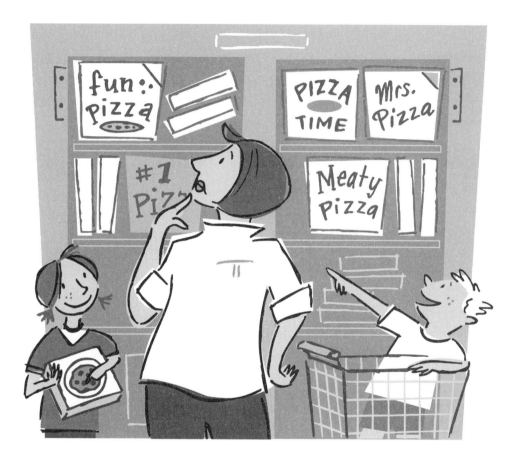

Do you ever wish there were 30 hours in a day? We do . . . especially on those hectic weeknights when we walk in the door and barely have enough time to preheat the oven. Can you say "frozen pizza tonight"? No-fuss convenience meals can save your neck when your family dinner hour looks more like 15 minutes. And what kid wouldn't be happy with a big bowl of mac & cheese or a hot dog and French fries for dinner?

But here's the catch. Not only are many frozen and boxed meals exceedingly high in sodium and saturated fat (and often trans fats), they also contain a long list of ingredients that most of us would be hard pressed to pronounce. In addition, many are also nutritional lightweights . . . providing little in the way of fiber, vitamins, minerals, and all those other powerful plant nutrients found in such things as fruits, vegetables, and whole grains.

The way we see it, if someone else is doing the cooking for you (and we don't mean a five-star chef), it's important to know what you're getting. But that's not so easy. In reality, it takes a lot of time to read and decipher all those food labels, not to mention taste every product to be sure the kids will even like it. That's where the Meal Makeover Moms come in. We've done the homework for you by evaluating the top ten convenience foods that busy moms feed their kids. We even used a panel of kid taste testers to help us out. Here's what we looked at: chicken nuggets, hot dogs, frozen pizza, boxed macaroni & cheese, frozen macaroni & cheese, frozen pot pies, frozen fish sticks, frozen burritos, frozen pocket sandwiches, and frozen French fries.

Anyone can give you a list of the so-called healthiest food products and brands on the market. But if they don't taste good and if your kids won't eat them, you're wasting your money. Here's what we considered when choosing the Best of the Bunch.

Moms' Best of the Bunch Criteria

KID APPEAL

If the majority of comments from our panel of kid taste testers was "yuck," "gross," or "do I have to eat this?" then the product was automatically disqualified (even if the Meal Makeover Moms were impressed with its nutritional profile).

INGREDIENTS

Any time you see an ingredient listed on a food label, rest assured the FDA considers it safe. That said, however, there are certain ingredients that we shy away from, including artificial colors, artificial flavors, monosodium glutamate (MSG), and nitrites. Will a food product containing any of these ingredients hurt you or your family? Probably not. But since some people, for instance, are sensitive to MSG and since some studies question the safety of eating a diet high in nitrites, we decided to look for brands without them.

FAT

When a frozen convenience product has 18 grams of saturated fat in a serving, you may want to leave it on the supermarket shelf. We consider 18 grams way too high given the fact that a person who consumes 2,000 calories a day is advised to keep their saturated fat intake below 20 grams. But you can't judge a food product by its saturated fat content alone. Many food products also contain trans fats (you may not see trans fat numbers on the labels just yet but you will by 2006). Like saturated fat, trans fats can also raise cholesterol levels and may be even worse for your heart. Foods made with shortening and/or partially hydrogenated vegetable oil contain trans fats . . . but unless you call the food company, you won't know how much. In order to qualify for the Best of the Bunch, a product had to therefore be low in both saturated fat and trans fats. While a food item wasn't automatically disqualified if shortening and/or hydrogenated oils appeared on the label, it certainly didn't help its chances.

SODIUM

If you're trying to limit your sodium intake to 2,400 milligrams a day (that's the current recommendation), then eating a convenience meal with half that amount is excessive. In general, we looked for Best of the Bunch winners with less than a third of the daily recommendation.

NUTRITIONAL SUPERSTARS

No one ever claimed a convenience meal could come anywhere close to Mom's home cooking but some may come closer than you'd think. In searching for our Best of the Bunch, we looked for products made with wholesome, all-natural ingredients such as nutrient-rich vegetables, plump chicken, real cheese, and whole grains.

Although we made sure that our choices for the Best of the Bunch were all national brands, it's possible your supermarket may not carry each and every one of them (don't forget to check the health food section of the supermarket as well). We encourage you to ask your store manager to consider stocking our suggested brands. Trust us, if enough shoppers request a particular food product, the supermarket will probably listen. Bear in mind too that products get reformulated. So even though we may have disqualified a certain item today doesn't mean it can't qualify for Best of the Bunch some time in the future. Our best advice is to read labels and visit our website on a regular basis for the latest product picks and pans. You can find us at *www.mealmakeovermoms.com*.

We hope as you cruise your local supermarket food aisles that you will use our Moms' Best of the Bunch criteria to find additional convenience foods that are just as wholesome, healthy, and flavorful as the products we list below. If you do, please tell us about them so we can share the news with other moms.

Chicken Nuggets

When a chicken nugget leaves a puddle of grease on your baking sheet or when you bite into one and wonder what that spongelike substance between the layers of breading really is, it may be time to start shopping for a new nugget. But don't despair, because we've done the legwork for you and are happy to report that there are several delicious and nutritious options out there that don't make you ponder "where's the chicken?"

Many of the popular chicken nugget products on the market contain a surprisingly modest amount of protein. That's too bad, since chicken meat is an excellent source of high-quality protein, a nutrient especially important for growing kids. To put protein in perspective, consider that our No-Nonsense Nuggets (page 276) contain 21 grams of protein in a 3-ounce serving while some of the frozen nuggets we found have 10 grams or less.

Besides nutrition (or lack thereof), there is also the issue of taste and texture. Here are just a few of the words used by our kid taste testers when sampling a dozen different brands of chicken nuggets: greasy, hollow, spongy, soggy, peppery, bland, cardboard, boring, salty, bready, and gross. As for their positive remarks on some of our Best of the Bunch brands: crunchy, real chicken, good flavor, and meaty.

MOMS' BEST OF THE BUNCH

With plenty of brands to choose from, it's clear people love chicken nuggets. The trick is in knowing which nuggets offer more than a mouthful of greasy breading (often made with hydrogenated oils). For the Best of the Bunch, we choose *Health is Wealth Chicken Nuggets, Ian's Chicken Nuggets, Bell & Evans Breaded Chicken Breast Nuggets* (the closest we found to homemade though a bit pricey), *Trader Joe's Chicken Drumettes,* and *Perdue Breaded Chicken Breast Nuggets.* Each can be found in the frozen food aisle with the exception of Perdue, located in the fresh meat aisle. All provide about 14 grams of protein and are made without hydrogenated oils (Perdue uses a small amount but the trans fats are negligible). As for their taste . . . our tasters give them "two thumbs up."

MOMS' QUICK FIX TIPS

- Dip in ketchup for a healthy dose of the antioxidant lycopene.
- Serve with any fruit or vegetable the kids are allowed to eat with their fingers: cherry or grape tomatoes, baby carrots, raw veggies and dip, grapes, blueberries, or sliced apples.
- Make chicken nuggets from scratch (see No-Nonsense Nuggets, page 276).

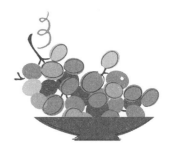

Hot Dogs

We call them hot dogs—you may know them as wieners or franks—but either way, there's no doubt that most people love them. In fact, Americans consume somewhere in the ballpark of 20 billion hot dogs each year! These days you can find all-beef, kosher, fat-free, veggie, chicken, turkey, even some dogs made with all-natural ingredients and no nitrites. What's a mom to do? With so many options, which are the best ones out there? Clearly, eating a hot dog with 350 calories, 990 milligrams of sodium, 32 grams of fat, and 15 grams of saturated fat is not the best nutritional choice. But neither is a fat-free frank with just 45 calories because hungry kids (and adults) need something a bit more substantial than that.

Personally, we don't mind a little bit of fat, but we do mind the sodium nitrite that most companies use in their hot dog products. Nitrites have come under fire over the years because some studies have linked the frequent consumption of nitrite-containing foods to a greater risk for certain cancers (one study looked at kids who ate twelve or more hot dogs a month and found a greater risk of childhood leukemia). Granted, if you eat an occasional hot dog, it's probably no big deal. But a regular diet of hot dogs along with things like bacon and luncheon meats (which can also contain nitrites) may not be prudent. Despite the possible health concerns, the FDA considers nitrites safe. Nitrites are used because they hinder the growth of bacteria and impart a cured flavor and pink color to the meat. While today, modern refrigeration keeps bacteria in check, companies continue to use nitrites, in part because consumers are accustomed to pink-colored franks.

MOMS' BEST OF THE BUNCH

It's not our intent to scare you or sensationalize a few diet studies. However, we figure it's a good idea to err on the side of caution when it comes to our kids' health. The good news is there are several delicious nitrite-free hot dogs on the market. Some are reddish in color (thanks to all-natural colorings) while others have more of a brownish-gray color. Get over it! Our Best of the Bunch are *Coleman All Natural Uncured Beef Hot Dogs, Hans' All Natural Uncured Beef Hot Dogs,* and *Applegate Farms Beef Hot Dogs.* All three remind us of the ballpark franks we ate as kids. The amount of saturated fat in each dog ranges from 2 to 4.5 grams, while the calories are anywhere from 100 to 140. Applegate Farms and a company called Wellshire Farms also make nitrite-free chicken dogs, so look for those as well. It's important to note that nitrite-free hot dogs are more perishable than traditional dogs. Once opened, place the uncooked leftovers in an airtight plastic bag and store in your refrigerator for three to four days, or you can just store them right away in your freezer.

- Serve on a whole wheat hot dog bun if available in your supermarket.
- Open a can of fiber-rich vegetarian baked beans and offer some on the side.
- Try one of the many nitrite-free vegetarian hot dogs on the market.

Frozen Vegetable Pizza

When we set out to evaluate all the frozen pizzas on the market, we soon realized that in order to taste each and every one of them, it would take weeks in the kitchen, not to mention indigestion that even our trusty bottles of Tums might never relieve. So instead of giving you the best of cheese, pepperoni, and sausage pizzas we decided to home in on vegetable pizzas instead, since they have the most potential for giving some balance to a meal. Our challenge was to straddle the fine line between a pizza with no vegetables at all and one with so many vegetables that most kids would get grossed out and refuse to eat it entirely.

Our pizza search revealed a wide range of choices. Some pies had little more than a sprinkling of green peppers, while others were loaded with an array of interesting veggies. We sampled pies with predictable toppings like bell peppers, mushrooms, onions, and olives but also found broccoli, spinach, shiitake mushrooms, bamboo shoots, sun-dried tomatoes, and artichoke hearts. As for the taste, well, that too was all across the board. One pizza, made with a whole wheat crust (unusual for a frozen pizza) turned out to be a bit too "healthy" for our young tasters. We had high hopes for this one but unfortunately, the crust didn't cut it.

Perhaps the biggest surprise of all was that we actually found ourselves rejecting a few of the most vegetable-laden pies. Don't get us wrong, folks, we love vegetables. But when big chunks of broccoli stalks are piled on high, trying to please young kids (who may freak when a vegetable touches their pizza) can become an even greater challenge.

MOMS' BEST OF THE BUNCH

We looked for a frozen veggie pizza with 6 grams or less of saturated fat, under 800 milligrams of sodium per serving, and a product made without hydrogenated vegetable oils. For our Best of the Bunch, we choose *Amy's Spinach, Veggie Combo,* and *Mushroom & Olive Pizzas, Trader Joe's Vegetarian Pizza,* and *Boca Rising Crust Pizza Supreme with Meatless Pepperoni & Sausage.* All have just the right amount of vegetables (not too few and not too many) in addition to all-natural ingredients. Our children also like *Stouffer's Grilled Vegetable French Bread Pizza.* Although it does have a small amount of trans fats, we appreciate the sweet red and yellow bell peppers and zucchini on top. Older children may appreciate the more sophisticated pizzas from A.C. LaRocco, such as *Tomato & Feta* and *Shiitake Mushroom*.

MOMS' QUICK FIX TIPS

- Stick to the suggested portion size to keep the calories and fat in check.
- If all you have is a frozen cheese pizza on hand, add your own veggies, such as sliced olives, artichoke hearts, bell pepper strips, or thawed frozen broccoli, or serve a salad or vegetable on the side.
- Make a veggie pizza from scratch (see Pizza Bonita, page 194).

Macaroni & Cheese in a Box

We really wish you could have been a fly on the wall the day we sampled all the boxed macaroni & cheese products from the market. Some were so "brightly colored," shall we say, that we needed our sunglasses to deflect the glare (okay . . . so maybe we're exaggerating just a bit). Since when is cheese supposed to be neon orange? Hey, we are all for eating a diet filled with colorful foods, but not when they're artificially colored with yellow 5 and yellow 6. Given the choice between a product with artificial ingredients or an all-natural brand, we would opt for the real thing every time.

If your kids are anything like ours, they probably love macaroni & cheese. And on nights when you don't have the time or inclination to make it from scratch (see page 172 for Fast-As-Boxed Macaroni & Cheese), what could be easier than opening a box? But keep in mind that there's more to mac & cheese than the noodles and cheese sauce alone. Don't forget about the half stick of butter or margarine that you add at the end or the nearly 20 grams of fat you get in each 1 cup serving.

MOMS' BEST OF THE BUNCH

When we see a food product with more ingredients than we can count on two hands or with names we can barely pronounce, we try to avoid it for the simple fact that we know other, more wholesome options are usually available. We therefore choose *Annie's Homegrown Shells & White Cheddar* and *Trader Joe's Macaroni & White Cheddar Cheese* for our Best of the Bunch. They are both made with natural ingredients such as pasta and Cheddar cheese and have a mild flavor kids love. We are also impressed with *Annie's Homegrown Whole Wheat Shells & Cheddar* with its 5 grams of fiber per serving, but admittedly, the whole wheat noodles are light brown in color, a fact that might put some kids off. But hey, you never know. The whole wheat is worth a try because it's really quite good.

- To reduce the saturated fat, prepare the macaroni & cheese with 2 tablespoons of olive oil and 1% lowfat milk instead of margarine or butter and whole milk.
- Add some extra protein and calcium by topping with chopped lean deli ham and preshredded reduced-fat Cheddar cheese.
- Stir in a can of flaked tuna fish and some frozen, thawed peas for a quick tuna noodle casserole.

Frozen Macaroni & Cheese

We think it's pretty ironic that of all the frozen macaroni & cheese products that we sampled, the one specifically marketed to kids (the fact that the pasta is shaped like little skateboards is a dead giveaway) has the highest amount of fat (17 grams) and sodium (1,160 milligrams) . . . making it the worst of the bunch. In all fairness, none of the products we tasted bowled us over in terms of taste or nutrition. Sure, most provide the same amount of bone-building calcium as a glass of milk, but given their bland taste and soggy texture, we're not sure it's worth the effort to turn on the oven.

Hey, this is just our humble opinion. Perhaps we're biased because we love the flavor, simplicity, and nutritional merits of our Fast-As-Boxed Macaroni & Cheese (page 172)—which, by the way, takes 20 minutes to prepare versus about 30 minutes to bake the frozen stuff.

MOMS' BEST OF THE BUNCH

We feel conflicted. We have to admit that we (and our kid tasters) really liked the flavor of *Amy's Macaroni & Cheese* as well as the fact that Amy's uses whole wheat flour in the pasta along with Cheddar cheese and other all-natural ingredients. But Amy's is higher in saturated fat than all the other brands. So in all fairness, we can't award it our Best of the Bunch (sob sob). That said, however, Amy's does make a frozen mac & cheese meal with soy cheese. *Amy's Macaroni & Soy Cheeze* has just 2 grams of saturated fat and is quite delicious. For our second winner, we choose *Stouffer's Lean Cuisine Macaroni & Cheese*. The ingredient list is longer than we would like, but within the frozen mac & cheese category, it has a nice flavor, no artificial colors, and only 4 grams of saturated fat.

MOMS' QUICK FIX TIPS

- Add more color to the meal by serving with bright colored vegetables (see Simply Delicious Broccoli, page 318).

- Mix in 2 tablespoons of salsa and $\frac{1}{3}$ cup frozen corn kernels, thawed, to kick up the flavor and round out the meal.
- Make mac & cheese from scratch (see Fast-As-Boxed Macaroni & Cheese, page 172).

Frozen Pot Pies

Imagine yourself walking down the frozen food aisle as you shop for a pot pie. Suddenly, you spot one with 7 grams of saturated fat . . . a number that looks pretty impressive next to some of the other pot pies with their 15 grams or more. But hold on, because numbers don't always tell the whole story. Also in that seemingly benign-looking pot pie you may find ingredients such as hydrogenated lard, partially hydrogenated soybean oil, and margarine . . . a clear indication the product contains trans fats. If you probe even further, it will quickly become clear that although the photo on the box shows a pie brimming with plump, juicy vegetables, what you are about to serve to your hungry child has just three puny peas, five little potato cubes, and a few tiny chunks of carrot.

The bottom line with pot pies is that most are high in calories, total fat, trans fats, sodium (the majority of those we evaluated had well over 800 milligrams in a serving), and in many cases, saturated fat. We were particularly unimpressed with one national brand with its 740 calories, 47 grams of fat, 18 grams of saturated fat, and 1,170 milligrams of sodium! Reading labels also indicates that the amount of vitamin A and vitamin C is often negligible—a tip-off that the product may have only a few gratuitous vegetables.

We'll grant you that a lot of these rich and flaky pot pies taste pretty darn good. But you can quickly lose your appetite when you begin to imagine just how much artery-clogging trans fats are lurking in each bite or when you read the ingredients label and see thirty-plus ingredients staring back at you. There's got to be a better way!

MOMS' BEST OF THE BUNCH

Given the fact that pot pies have a flaky pie crust on the bottom and the top makes it difficult to find a lot of healthy options out there, our best advice is to therefore limit your family's consumption. But when you must have pot pie (and sometimes you just must), go with *Amy's Broccoli Pot Pie with Cheddar Cheese Sauce* for the Best of the Bunch. This delicious, all-natural pot pie is filled with a colorful mix of broccoli, carrots, and potatoes as well as 100% real Cheddar cheese.

It is a bit higher in saturated fat than we would like because the crust contains some butter and the company uses full-fat cheese versus lowfat. But we feel okay about Amy's for a few important reasons: First, each pie offers a day's worth of vitamin A and nearly 50 percent of the vitamin C, thanks to all those healthy vegetables. Second, it is made with real ingredients, including high-fiber whole wheat flour. And finally, there are no hydrogenated oils or shortening used in the crust, making this product trans fat free.

If you prefer a pot pie with chicken, then go with *Shelton's Pot Pie*. It's made with an all natural whole wheat crust and has 5 grams of saturated fat . . . making it one of the Best of the Bunch.

MOMS' QUICK FIX TIPS

- Cook up some frozen mixed vegetables and serve them alongside the pie. They'll get smothered with the saucy filling and blend right in.
- Eat the crispy top half of the pie crust but leave the soggy bottom crust behind.
- Serve with a glass of lowfat milk, since pot pies contain little in the way of calcium.

Frozen Fish Sticks

When you see the word "fish," you automatically think: "healthy." And why not? Fish is naturally low in saturated fat and contains healthy omega-3 fatty acids. But when you take fish, coat it in a breading mixture made with hydrogenated oils, sprinkle some MSG on top, and then deep-fat fry it, your catch of the day misses the boat when it comes to good nutrition.

We had to cast a wide net to find a fish stick product that we, in good conscience, could feed our children and recommend for yours. Some of the fish sticks we found were made with hydrogenated oils but contained less than 1 gram of trans fats (nothing to lose sleep over), but others had a boat-load. Since labels may not yet list trans fat information, we figure if you can find a delicious fish stick made with canola oil or soybean oil, then you might as well go for it. It's worth noting that we did find two products with very little fat (2.5 grams per serving), but they were so bland and dry that no one liked them.

Fish sticks aren't exactly cool with older teens, but for the younger school-age crowd, they're a great last-minute standby. Moms love them for their simplicity . . . kids love them for their crunch.

MOMS' BEST OF THE BUNCH

Eating fish sticks will never come anywhere close to a dinner of grilled salmon. But on those hectic nights when you're too tired to fire up the grill, fish sticks can save the day. For our Best of the Bunch we choose *Natural Sea Fish Sticks, Trader Joe's Cod Sticks,* and *Ian's Lightly Breaded Fish Sticks*. All contain 6 to 10 grams of total fat, only 1 gram of saturated fat, no trans fats, and just a little bit of sodium. Extra credit goes to Natural Sea for their use of whole wheat flour in the breading, a contribution of 2 grams of fiber.

- Create your own healthy tartar sauce by mixing together $\frac{1}{4}$ cup light canola mayonnaise, 1 tablespoon relish, 1 tablespoon ketchup, and $\frac{1}{2}$ teaspoon lemon juice.
- Serve with a vegetable that's shaped like a stick: green beans, asparagus, carrot sticks.
- Make fish sticks from scratch (see Flaky Fish Sticks, page 248).

Burritos

Burritos sound healthy, and in many cases, they are. Our favorites come loaded with wholesome ingredients like pinto beans, black beans, vegetables, brown rice, soy cheese, and regular cheese, and range in flavor from mild to hot and spicy. They're typically a good source of protein and fiber and, with a salad on the side, can be a meal in and of themselves. But you can also get burned in the frozen food aisle like we did when we picked up a seemingly healthy chicken burrito. Although the label indicated only 1 gram of saturated fat, when we cut it open, a strange, pastelike substance came oozing out. Even Janice's husband, Don (who eats just about anything you put in front of him), refused to take a bite. Besides its appearance and aroma, the fact that the product also contained chicken fat, mechanically separated chicken, and partially hydrogenated vegetable oil motivated us to move on to the next product.

Making your own homemade burritos is a breeze, but on those nights when you're out of flour tortillas or just too tired to open a can of beans, nothing could be easier than heating a frozen burrito in the microwave or oven.

MOMS' BEST OF THE BUNCH

If your family has been asking for more vegetarian meals, then burritos can come to your rescue, as many are made with beans and no meat. For our Best of the Bunch, we choose *Cedarlane Organic Roasted Vegetable & Cheese Burrito, Cedarlane Beans, Rice, & Cheese Style Burrito, Amy's Organic Beans & Rice Burrito, Trader Joe's Grilled Vegetable & Black Bean Burrito* (if your kids don't like onions, try another one), and *Trader Joe's Mildly Spiced Vegetable Burrito* (the spiciest of them all). All have 3 grams of saturated fat or less.

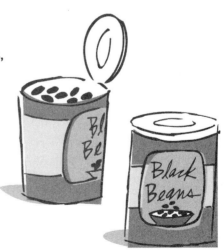

- Serve with a glass of orange juice or dip in salsa. Those vitamin C–rich foods will enhance the absorption of iron from all the beans.
- Open a bag of prewashed greens and make a quick salad.
- Make burritos from scratch (see Colorful Sweet Potato Burritos, page 128).

Frozen Pocket Sandwiches

You can't walk down the frozen food aisle these days without noticing all those convenient hand-held, grab-and-go sandwich pockets. With flavors like cheeseburger, meatballs and mozzarella, and Philly steak and cheese, they're so popular that one company alone sells well over $500 million dollars' worth each year . . . and that's not pocket change!

When we set out to evaluate sandwich pockets, we thought it would be fairly easy to weed out the Best of the Bunch. After all, there are plenty of "lean" options to choose from out there. Take, for example, a "lean" pocket made with chicken, Cheddar, and broccoli. A label comparison shows that the "lean" version has half the fat and saturated fat of its regular, full-fat counterpart. But as we have learned, you can't judge a product by the numbers alone. For starters, the ingredients listed on that so-called "lean" chicken pocket reveal such things as margarine and hydrogenated soybean and cottonseed oil . . . a clue the product also contains trans fats. "Okay," you may be thinking, "what's the big deal if the pocket has some trans fats . . . don't all those bright green broccoli florets featured on the package more than make up for it?" Well, ladies, we thought the same thing, but when we actually cooked the pocket, we needed a magnifying glass and a pair of tweezers to find the scant teaspoon or two of broccoli bits sealed up within. In all honesty, we had a hunch there wasn't going to be too much broccoli inside since vitamins A and C were not even listed on the label.

Even though pockets are often considered a small meal or snack, they can still offer an opportunity to weave a bit of good nutrition into your family's diet. Unfortunately, a lot of the popular pockets offer little in the way of vegetables and sometimes even include "imitiation" cheese and artificial colors and flavors. Let the search begin!

MOMS' BEST OF THE BUNCH

There is only so much you can fit into a pocket, so expectations should not be too high. That said, however, we choose *Amy's Broccoli & Cheese in a Pocket Sandwich, Amy's Cheese Pizza in a Pocket Sandwich,* and *Applegate Farms Cheese Pepperoni Pizza Hand Held Stuffed Sandwich* as our Best of the Bunch. All three taste great and are made with all-natural ingredients as well as real cheese. Bear in mind that the Applegate pepperoni pocket is a bit spicy and may therefore be more appealing to older children or kids who like hot food.

MOMS' QUICK FIX TIPS

- If you're on the run, serve with some grab-and-go fruits or vegetables such as grapes, apples, baby carrots, or bananas.
- If you're eating at home, serve with a bowl of vegetable soup or tomato soup or a big green salad.
- Make a pocket from scratch (see Quick Quesadilla Pockets, page 198).

Helpful Web Sites

If you have trouble finding any of our Best of the Bunch picks in your local super-market, check out the company web sites. There, you can find out which supermarkets across the country carry each product.

A.C. LaRocco: www.aclarocco.com

Amy's Kitchen: www.amyskitchen.com

Annie's Homegrown: www.annies.com

Applegate Farms: www.applegatefarms.com

Alexia Foods: www.alexiafoods.com

Bell & Evans: www.bellandevans.com

Boca Foods: www.bocaburger.com

Cascadian Farm: www.cfarm.com

Cedarlane Natural Foods: www.cedarlanefoods.com

Coleman Natural Beef: www.colemanmeats.com

Hans' All Natural: www.hansallnatural.com

Health is Wealth Foods: www.healthiswealthfoods.com

Ian's Natural Foods: www.iansnaturalfoods.com

Shelton's: www.sheltons.com

Trader Joe's: www.traderjoes.com

Wellshire Farms: www.wellshirefarms.com

Frozen French Fries

When we set out to review frozen French fries we had a hunch that most would be high in fat, loaded with sodium, and made with partially hydrogenated vegetable oils, and that's exactly what we found. But never in our wildest dreams did we ever imagine we would encounter a frozen French fry with the brightest turquoise blue color we'd ever seen. After digesting the fact that some kids actually eat blue French fries, we spotted another product—this one chocolate-flavored—with the equivalent of 5 teaspoons of sugar in each 3-ounce serving. Wow! The French fry market has sure come a long way since we were kids.

French fries occupy a huge chunk of the supermarket frozen food aisle. There, you'll find taters and tots, steak fries and curly fries, sweet potato fries, cheese fries, even purple fries (those, by the way, are made from purple potatoes). It's easy to see why potatoes are America's most popular vegetable. Potatoes are naturally fat free and considered a good source of vitamin C. But when they're processed into French fries, not only do they lose most of their vitamin C, they also gain a hefty dose of fat.

MOMS' BEST OF THE BUNCH

Before we even began our evaluation of frozen French fries, we were excited to try some of the sweet potato fries on the market, given their stellar nutritional profile. To our disappointment, however, most didn't crisp up in the oven and were not well accepted by our children. Sweet potato fries are worth a try, but don't expect that crisp-on-the-outside, tender-on-the-inside characteristic of most French fries. For our Best of the Bunch, we stick with good old-fashioned fries. We choose *Ian's Alphatots* and *Quick Fries, Cascadian Farm French Fries, Alexia Trio Fries,* and *Alexia Yukon Gold Julienne Fries.* All are made with oils that have not been hydrogenated. We also love the flavor of *Ian's Cheddar Cheese Fries* and *Cascadian Farm Spud Puppies,* though both are higher in sodium than we would like. Honorable mention goes to *Ore-Ida Golden Crinkles.* We like the taste and although they contain a small amount of trans fats, it's less than most of the other mainstream brands on the market.

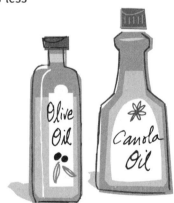

MOMS' QUICK FIX TIPS

- Serve another vegetable with the meal, because French fries offer little in the way of vitamins A and C.
- Dip in ketchup for a healthy dose of lycopene, an antioxidant that may lower cancer risk.
- Make French fries from scratch (see Sweet Potato Fries, page 304).

Fast Food Fix

Some might argue that the ultimate convenience foods can be found at the drive-thru window at any number of fast food establishments dotting every highway, byway, and strip mall in America. While we agree that fast food is ultra convenient, eating it on a regular basis can sabotage your family's meal makeover. Sure, fast food restaurants now offer some healthy options, but we can't let them off the hook so easily. It's important to know that fast food companies spend a lot of time, effort, and money marketing their food to your children and competing for your dollar. Consider the fact that fast food chains spend a staggering $3 billion annually on TV advertising alone. The returns are huge. In 2001, Americans spent $110 billion on fast food.

Brand loyalty begins when children are as young as the age of two. So you'd better believe that fast food companies make a big effort to introduce their products, logos, and jingles to your children early on. Visit their web sites and you'll know what we mean. For example, if you go to Burger King's web site, you'll notice a link for the Big Kids Club. And what kid wouldn't beg his mom to join after reading the following: "There's a ton of free loot in it for you. I'm talkin' a free hamburger meal on your birthday— and other awesome stuff like screensavers, 3-D pictures and funny jokes. It's all FREE!" The club may be free, but the amount of calories, fat, sugar, and sodium in one of their Big Kids meals certainly is not. Order a Big Kids meal complete with a double cheeseburger, small fries, and a 16-ounce soft drink and we're talkin' 940 calories, 42 grams of fat, 12 teaspoons of sugar, and 1,595 milligrams of sodium.

In our opinion, when it comes to fast food, the best nutritional scenario would be not to eat it at all. Just drive by the drive-thru. Since prohibiting fast food altogether, however, may not be feasible for many families, a goal of fewer visits may be more realistic. But limiting your visits is just one way to fix fast food.

ORDER UP SOME INFORMATION

Which has more fat, calories, and sodium? A McDonald's Filet-O-Fish sandwich or a McDonald's Quarter Pounder? If you guessed the Quarter Pounder, you're wrong. Surprisingly, the fish sandwich has more of all of the above. Ordering fish or chicken instead of beef doesn't guarantee a healthier fast food meal. And don't assume that the "healthy" salad options are necessarily low in fat and sodium either. At one fast food restaurant, a Crispy Chicken California Cobb Salad with a packet of Ranch Dressing has 53 grams of fat and 1,700 milligrams of sodium (order the light dressing and your sodium shoots up to 2,120 milligrams). That's why it's critical that you arm yourself with as much nutrition information as possible so you can make the best, most informed choices. Many fast food restaurants now display nutritional information on all of their menu items. If it's not posted, ask for it. You can also visit many fast food companies' web sites and view the numbers there. Some web sites even allow you to select different menu items to create a virtual meal that is then nutritionally analyzed for you. Don't forget that food products are constantly reformulated while new ones are added, so be on the lookout for updated information.

DOWNSIZE . . . DON'T SUPERSIZE

Fast food restaurants are notorious for their larger-than-life food and beverage portions. There, you can find Super Size French fries, 42-ounce soft drinks, Ultimate Cheeseburgers, and 32-ounce Triple Thick Shakes. With larger portions, people feel like they're getting more for their money. Unfortunately, in many cases they are . . . more calories, more artery-clogging saturated and trans fats, and more sodium. Bear in mind that a person who consumes 2,000 calories a day should limit her saturated fat intake to less than 20 grams and sodium to less than 2,400 milligrams.

Look how a simple switch from a supersized portion to a smaller one can dramatically cut calories and saturated fat.

SUPERSIZE (BEFORE)	DOWNSIZE (AFTER)
32-ounce McDonald's Chocolate Triple Thick Shake (1,150 calories, 22 g saturated fat)	12-ounce McDonald's Chocolate Triple Thick Shake (430 calories, 8 g saturated fat)
McDonald's Super Size French Fries (610 calories, 5 g saturated fat)	McDonald's Small French Fries (210 calories, 1.5 g saturated fat)
Taco Bell Grilled Stuft Beef Burrito (730 calories, 11 g saturated fat)	Taco Bell Fiesta Steak Burrito (370 calories, 4 g saturated fat)
Burger King Original Double Whopper with Cheese (1,150 calories, 30 g saturated fat)	Burger King Cheeseburger (360 calories, 8 g saturated fat)
Arby's Big Montana (630 calories, 15 g saturated fat)	Arby's Regular Roast Beef (350 calories, 6 g saturated fat)

SMART SWAPS

Fast food has a bad reputation, and it's easy to see why. Eating a Whopper with Cheese, large fries, medium soft drink, and a piece of pie for dessert contributes a whopping 1,953 calories, 96 grams of fat, 30 grams of saturated fat, 10 grams of trans fats, and 2,786 milligrams of sodium to the

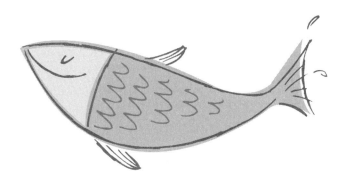

diet. Making smart swaps at the fast food window or counter can shave more than just calories from your fast food meal . . . and with little effort.

The following chart highlights just a few examples for improving your fast food choices. To make other healthy swaps, simply check out the nutrition information posted at your fast food restaurant. And don't forget, you can always have it your way if you request one of the following: a kid's meal with lowfat milk instead of a soft drink, a sandwich with lowfat mayo or ketchup instead of the high-fat sauces and spreads, or a burger, chicken, or fish sandwich with lettuce and tomato.

Go Out of the Box

Nothing says you have to order a burger, fries, and shake every time you stop by your local fast food restaurant. Try going "out of the box" by choosing less traditional menu items that are just as quick but don't provide a day's worth of fat, calories, and sodium in one sitting. Try some of the following diamonds in the rough:

- Burger King Veggie Burger (300 calories, 10 g fat, 1.5 g saturated fat, 770 mg sodium). *Bonus:* 4 g fiber, 35% iron.
- Wendy's Hot Stuffed Broccoli & Cheese Potato (480 calories, 14 g fat, 3 g saturated fat, 510 mg sodium). *Bonus:* 35% vitamin A, 120% vitamin C, 20% calcium.
- KFC Mean (collard) Greens (70 calories, 3 g fat, 1 g saturated fat, 650 mg sodium). *Bonus:* 60% vitamin A, 10% vitamin C, 20% calcium, 5 g fiber.
- McDonald's Fruit 'n Yogurt Parfait with Granola (380 calories, 5 g fat, 2 g saturated fat, 240 mg sodium). *Bonus:* 40% vitamin C, 40% calcium.
- Chick-fil-A Carrot & Raisin Salad (130 calories, 5 g fat, 1 g saturated fat, 90 mg sodium). *Bonus:* 170% vitamin A, 2 g fiber.

INSTEAD OF THIS . . .	CHOOSE THIS . . .	AND ELIMINATE . . .
McDonald's Spanish Omelet Bagel	McDonald's Egg McMuffin	410 calories 10 g saturated fat 680 mg sodium
McDonald's Big Mac	McDonald's Cheeseburger	260 calories 5 g saturated fat 270 mg sodium
Burger King Whopper Jr.	Burger King Chicken Whopper Jr.	150 calories 9 g saturated fat 155 mg sodium
KFC Chunky Chicken Pot Pie	KFC Tender Roast Sandwich Corn on the Cob Cole Slaw	280 calories 10.5 g saturated fat 1,240 mg sodium *Bonus:* Triple the fiber
2 slices Pizza Hut Stuffed Crust Pepperoni Lover's Pizza	2 slices Pizza Hut Thin 'n Crispy Veggie Lover's Pizza	460 calories 12 g saturated fat 1,660 mg sodium *Bonus:* Vitamin C
Taco Bell Taco Salad with Salsa	Taco Bell Taco Salad with Salsa without Shell	370 calories 21 g total fat 270 mg sodium
16-ounce "small" soft drink	12-ounce orange juice	10 calories 3 teaspoons sugar *Bonus:* 160% vitamin C
Mayonnaise	Ketchup	145 calories 2.5 g saturated fat *Bonus:* Lycopene
Dunkin Donuts Coffee Cake Muffin	Dunkin Donuts Wheat Bagel with $\frac{1}{2}$ packet lite cream cheese	295 calories 4.5 g saturated fat 12 teaspoons sugar *Bonus:* Double the fiber
Wendy's house vinaigrette dressing	Wendy's lowfat honey mustard dressing	100 calories 3 g saturated fat 460 mg sodium

ON THE ROAD AGAIN

When you're on a road trip with the kids, you have few options when stomachs start to growl. Or do you? Instead of the inevitable fast food pit stop, fill a cooler with things like bottled water, juice boxes, baby carrots, cheese sticks, peanut butter and jelly sandwiches, raisins, grapes, sliced apples, and animal crackers and offer a snack or meal along the way. Sometimes it's more fun to stop at a rest area or park where you can stretch your legs, play ball, and have a picnic rather than being stuck at an anonymous fast food joint. Being prepared can save you money and hundreds of calories to boot.

CHAPTER 4

The Meal Makeover Pantry

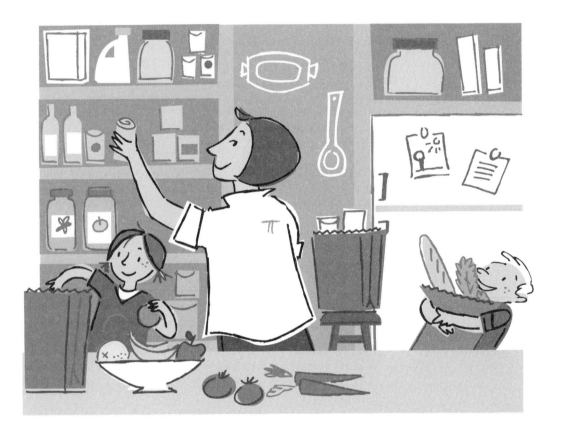

The foods you stock in your kitchen cupboards, refrigerator, and freezer (aka the pantry) can make or break your family's meal makeover. That's why our Meal Makeover Pantry is brimming with foods that help to weave super nutrition into everything you eat. As an added bonus, the items we recommend are also designed to get you in and out of the kitchen in as little time as possible without compromising great flavor. Our pantry items are not exotic or out of the ordinary because what Meal Makeover Moms like you really need are the basics. Let's face it. If many of us were to open up our kitchen cupboards right now, we'd probably find bottles of gourmet marinades and sauces that we "had to buy" but never once opened. Blow off the dust and read on.

Today's busy moms have to compete with the convenience of fast food, frozen meals, and take-out. And since there is typically so little free time in the day, moms often lose the battle. That's why we believe it's essential to fill your pantry with shortcut ingredients such as canned beans, salsa, frozen vegetables, pasta, canned tuna, preshredded carrots, and other staples that help to get meals on the table quickly. While we have nothing against convenience meals when chosen wisely, with a well-stocked pantry, you have plenty of other options. For example, with the help of preshredded cheese, in 20 minutes flat, you can make your own macaroni & cheese from scratch with twice the protein and calcium of the boxed stuff. Using our pantry items, you can also whip up your own chicken nuggets (with real chicken meat . . . imagine that!), pizza, tacos, hot sandwich pockets, alphabet soup, quesadillas, chocolate pudding, and much, much more.

Our pantry is designed to entice taste buds of all ages with new flavors, textures, and taste sensations. If your children aren't big fans of cooked vegetables, you can kick up the flavor by drizzling extra virgin olive oil and a pinch of kosher salt or a lowfat cheese sauce over the top. We have other flavor tricks in our pantry as well. You can add raisins and sunflower seeds to coleslaw for sweetness and crunch, incorporate shredded carrots into soups and sandwiches for subtle sweetness, and use savory chopped nuts for breadings and toppings in place of the usual bread crumbs.

Last, but not least, our Meal Makeover Pantry helps to improve the nutritional GPA of your family's diet. Our idea of good nutrition does not include fat-free cottage cheese or sour cream, foods "sautéed" in nonstick cooking spray, thin-sliced "diet" breads, salt-free soups and broths, egg substitutes, or fat-free cookies. In other words, we're not about deprivation. What we are about is real foods that taste great and come naturally packed with nutrients that promote good health. Therefore, what you'll find in our pantry are things like olive oil and canola oil, rich in healthy fats; canned beans, an inexpensive source of protein and fiber; and wheat germ, a vitamin E booster that makes its way into delicious recipes like our Blueberry Banana Pancakes (page 152) and our Banana Chocolate Chip Muffins (page 340). One of our favorite pantry "must-haves" is frozen vegetables. Before you gasp at such nutritional blasphemy, you'll be happy to know that frozen can actually be more nutritious than fresh. Indeed, frozen vegetables are indispensable, especially when you're out of the fresh kind.

Even on the busiest nights of the week when you're in one of those all-too-familiar multitasking modes (you know, helping the kids with their homework, answering phone calls from pushy telemarketers, and feeding the family pet), it's possible to create nourishing meals that everyone will enjoy. The good news is you don't have to be a great cook or even one of those supermoms who always manages to whip up fabulous meals from virtually nothing. Our pantry will inspire you to prepare easy meals—with or without a recipe—with whatever happens to be on hand.

The Meal Makeover Moms' Kitchen Cupboard

The time has finally come to roll up your sleeves and reorganize your kitchen cabinets. If you've been putting this off for years or even decades, don't delay, because when you get right down to it, this should only take a couple of hours. It might actually be kind of fun. Mom gets to make a mess for a change!

The reason we want you to clean off your pantry shelves is because, chances are, you have no idea what's hiding behind those boxes of dried pasta and cans of baked beans. It's funny how certain items get shoved to the back of the cupboard and linger there well beyond their expiration dates. If you don't know what's in your pantry, you can't use it as a tool for getting fast and healthy meals to your table night after night.

Once you've discarded all those things that are no longer edible and those you can't even identify, you can begin the process of reorganizing and restocking. Now is the time to make room for new things that may have never been in your kitchen before: whole wheat pasta and couscous, whole wheat flour, bulgur, salmon in a can or pouch, canned pure pumpkin, kosher salt, and cartons of all-natural chicken or vegetable broth to name just a few. When you put things back on your pantry shelves, be sure to assign a specific place for each food category, including one for canned beans, dried pasta, canned meats, pasta sauces, rice . . . you get the picture. That way when you go to grab a can of black beans for your Last-Minute Black Bean Soup (page 106), you'll know exactly where to look. Your days of fishing around blindly in the back of a dark cupboard are over.

COOKING OILS

As Meal Makeover Moms, we are committed to good flavor and good health, which is why cooking oils are found front and center in our pantry. Certain cooking oils contain beneficial monounsaturated fats and omega-3 polyunsaturated fats. By no means are we advocating deep-fat frying. But we do want you to know that a tablespoon here or a drizzle there can certainly jazz up your meals. There is no shortage of cooking oils to choose from these days . . . with everything from familiar oils like vegetable and corn to the more gourmet macadamia nut and walnut oils. To keep life simple, for the most part, we tend to cook (and drizzle) with the following:

Canola Oil: This mild-flavored vegetable oil is low in saturated fat and a good source of monounsaturated fats and omega-3 fats. It works well in baking, sautéing, and for oiling pans.

Olive Oil: Extra virgin olive oil has a deep, almost fruity flavor that varies from brand to brand. It's ideal for salad dressings and drizzling over cooked vegetables or slices of French bread. Pure (virgin) and light olive oils are milder in flavor, hold up better under high heat, and are best for sautéing and baking. Both contain mainly monounsaturated fats.

Peanut Oil and Toasted Sesame Oil: These oils are highly flavored and ideal for Asian-style dishes. Peanut oil holds up well under high heat so we often use it in stir-fries (check out our Mixed-Up Tofu, page 204).

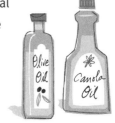

Nonstick Cooking Spray: We would never use nonstick cooking spray to sauté a piece of chicken but it certainly comes in handy when coating baking pans and muffin tins. Look for a nonstick spray made with canola or olive oil.

Tip: In general, the shelf life of cooking oil is 3 to 12 months. To keep your oils from turning rancid once they've been opened, store them in a cool, dark place. You can also keep cooking oils in your refrigerator. While this may turn them cloudy, it won't affect their flavor or quality.

CONDIMENTS AND DRESSINGS

Imagine a hamburger without ketchup or a tuna sandwich without mayo. Boring! Condiments and dressings can add the final exclamation point to a meal. But beware, because some can bring excessive amounts of calories, fat, and sodium to your table.

Mayonnaise: One-quarter cup of full-fat mayonnaise has 400 calories and 44 grams of fat while light mayo has half that amount. While we don't usually get too uptight about fat (unless of course it's the saturated or trans fat kind), given the fact that more than half of our country's population is overweight, we suggest a lower-calorie version for most people. Look for a mayonnaise made with canola oil. We use *Cains Light* and *Spectrum Lite Canola Mayo.*

Salad Dressings: Whether you choose a full-fat, reduced-fat, light, or fat-free salad dressing is entirely up to you. But remember that the calories in regular salad dressings can quickly add up (2 tablespoons of ranch dressing have 160 calories and 17 grams of fat) so if you're watching your weight, a reduced-fat option may be better.

Mustard: Use honey and Dijon mustards for added flavor with minimal calories.

Ketchup: We give ketchup two thumbs up. Sure, it contains some sugar and salt, but if ketchup entices your kids to eat healthy foods, using a small amount can go a long way. Ketchup is also a great source of lycopene, a cancer-fighting antioxidant.

Salsa: Some like it hot . . . but watch out, because certain brands contain mucho sodium. Look for a salsa with less than 175 milligrams of sodium per serving (2 tablespoons). You can add salsa to just about anything. We use it to kick up the flavor in our Turkey All Wrapped Up (page 141), Mexican Lasagna (page 228), and Southwestern Chicken & Rice (page 292).

Real Bacon Bits: Bacon bits can be very high in sodium but a small amount imparts a lot of flavor . . . and you know what, we can't be perfect all the time, now can we? Beware of imitation bacon bits, because some contain artificial colors, flavors, and all sorts of other yucky stuff.

Vinegar: Balsamic vinegar, rice vinegar, red wine vinegar, and white wine vinegar add a flavor kick without the calories.

ETHNIC FLAVOR ENHANCERS

Our favorite ethnic flavor enhancers include soy sauce, teriyaki sauce, oyster sauce, Thai peanut sauce, and hoisin sauce. In general, they are very salty. In fact, oyster sauce can have as much as 1,000 milligrams of sodium in 1 tablespoon alone. But don't despair, because you really don't need to use a whole lot to bring big flavors to your cooking. Just check out our recipe for Hunan Beef & Broccoli (page 224) and you'll see what we mean. Some sauces are available in lighter versions with 50 percent less sodium. If you are sensitive to monosodium glutamate (MSG), read labels and choose a product that's MSG free. We use *Kikkoman Lite Soy Sauce* and *Kikkoman Lite Teriyaki*.

CANNED FOODS

Canned foods don't always get the respect they deserve. But if you cook dinner night after night, canned foods can make your job easier and your meals a lot more nutritious. For example, if your family loves beef tacos, consider adding a can of black beans to the beef mixture (see Have-It-Your-Way Tacos, page 234). You'll double the fiber and add other nutrients as well. All it takes is a can opener and 20 extra seconds at the kitchen counter. It's that easy!

Canned Fruit: Canned fruit packed in water or its own natural juices has half the calories of fruit packed in syrup. Keep canned fruits such as Mandarin oranges, pineapple, and pears on hand for quick snacks and for using in your recipes. You'll love the flavor that canned pineapple brings to our Sweet & Slightly Sour Shrimp (page 262).

Canned Vegetables: A lot of us grew up eating canned corn and canned peas, but there's a world of other canned vegetables to choose from. We wouldn't be without canned pumpkin, sweet

The Trouble with MSG

Monosodium glutamate (MSG) is widely used around the world to enhance the flavor of meats, soups, seasonings, snack foods, frozen convenience meals, sauces, and much, much more. Some people complain of adverse reactions to MSG, ranging from nausea and vomiting to migraine headaches and heart palpitations. If you or someone in your family is sensitive to MSG, read labels carefully. Be aware that other commonly used ingredients may contain monosodium glutamate, including hydrolyzed vegetable protein, autolyzed yeast, glutamate, and textured vegetable protein.

potatoes, hominy (the secret ingredient in our Halftime Taco Chili, page 120), baby corn, and artichoke hearts.

Canned Beans: Stock your pantry with canned black beans, kidney beans, pinto beans, black-eyed peas, cannellini beans (white beans), and chickpeas. They're packed with fiber and nutrients. Canned beans can be salty, so be sure to drain and rinse them before adding them to a dish. Believe it or not, rinsing beans can remove 30 to 40 percent of the sodium. If you think your family won't like canned beans, you'll be surprised how versatile and flavorful they can be. Liz's boys both love the pinto beans in our Confetti Chicken Wraps (page 278).

Refried Beans: Refried beans are often made with lard, so stock your pantry with a fat-free brand to eliminate the saturated fat but not the flavor. Turn to our Wrap & Roll ideas (page 000) for a clever way to add refried beans to your dinner menu.

Canned Fish: Canned baby shrimp, minced clams, tuna, and skinless, boneless salmon are ultra convenient when there are slim pickins at the seafood counter. As an added bonus, all contain healthy omega-3 fats. You can also find tuna and salmon packaged in shelf-stable pouches.

Tip: Canned tuna packed in water has about half the calories of tuna packed in oil.

SOUPS AND BROTHS

Canned soups, broths, and bouillon cubes are all over the board when it comes to nutrition. Most are extraordinarily high in sodium and a surprising number contain monosodium glutamate. The good news is, however, that plenty of healthier soup and broth options exist in today's supermarkets, including those made with all-natural ingredients as well as less sodium, saturated fat, and trans fats.

Canned Soups: There are oodles of options in the canned soup aisle. It gets kind of confusing after a while. Given all the choices—fat-free, reduced-sodium, all-natural, organic, and healthy—it's hard to know what's best for your family. Our most important word of advice is to read labels carefully. Here's why: You would think that a can of Campbell's Cream of Mushroom Soup, touted as "98% fat free," would be the healthiest one on the shelf. But after reading the label, you quickly discover that each serving has 3 grams of fat (not too bad), 900 milligrams of sodium (too high), and MSG to boot. For comparison, if you look at Campbell's Healthy Request Cream of Mushroom Soup, you'll find less fat, half the sodium, and no MSG at all. Another reason to read labels is that some soups contain a significant amount of vitamins A and C, a clear indication they're packed with vegetables. For example, a can of Health Valley Lentil & Carrot soup (something we use in our Shells with Soupy Lentil Sauce, page 214) provides 80 percent of the RDA of vitamin A per serving while a can of the more popular Progresso Lentil soup has just 15 percent in a serving. Why miss an opportunity to get more vegetables into your family's diet? We use *Health Valley, Amy's Organic,* and *Campbell's Healthy Request* soups.

If You Can Boil Water...You Can Make Dinner

Have you ever noticed how some moms have a real knack for grabbing a can of this and a jar of that and then creating an amazing meal, even without a recipe? Don't you just hate them? Well, we decided to show you how easy it can be to improvise with the ingredients in your new Meal Makeover Pantry. We devised three "throw it together" meal ideas that start with a pot of boiling water. If time is not on your side, be sure to put that pot of water on the stove and crank up the heat the minute you walk in the door (in other words, before you feed the dog or read the mail).

Shrimp Teriyaki Noodles (Serves 5)

PANTRY ITEMS NEEDED:

Medium egg noodles (8 ounces, about 4 cups)

Frozen broccoli florets, thawed (16-ounce bag)

Peanut oil (1 tablespoon)

Frozen precooked small or medium shrimp, thawed (16-ounce bag)

Lite teriyaki sauce ($1/3$ cup)

Water ($1/3$ cup)

Lite soy sauce (1 tablespoon)

Cornstarch (2 teaspoons)

QUICK FIX:

Bring a big saucepan of water to a boil. Add the noodles and cook according to package directions. A few minutes before they're done, toss in the broccoli. Bring the water back to a boil and cook until the pasta and broccoli are cooked to your liking. Drain and set aside. Return the empty saucepan to the stove, add the oil, and heat over medium-high heat. Add the shrimp and sauté 1 to 2 minutes. Meanwhile, whisk together the teriyaki sauce, water, soy sauce, and cornstarch. Once the shrimp are hot, add the well-blended teriyaki sauce mixture to the pan and stir for a minute or two until it thickens. Now add the broccoli and pasta back to the pan, mix everything together, heat through, and you're good to go. For added flavor and crunch, top with chopped peanuts.

Creamy Macaroni & Salmon (Serves 4)

PANTRY ITEMS NEEDED:

Small elbow macaroni (8 ounces, about 2 cups)

Skinless, boneless pink salmon (7-ounce pouch or 6-ounce can)

Frozen green peas, thawed ($1\frac{1}{2}$ cups)

Reduced-fat sour cream ($\frac{2}{3}$ cup)

Preshredded reduced-fat Cheddar cheese ($\frac{2}{3}$ cup)

Grated Parmesan cheese ($\frac{1}{3}$ cup)

QUICK FIX:

Bring a big saucepan of water to a boil. Add the pasta and cook according to package directions. Drain and immediately return to the pan. Add the salmon (be sure to flake it first), peas, sour cream, Cheddar cheese, and Parmesan cheese. Mix everything together, heat through, and serve.

Mega Minestrone (Serves 4)

PANTRY ITEMS NEEDED:

Dried ditalini pasta (4 ounces, about 1 cup)

Frozen mixed vegetables, thawed (2 cups)

Ready-to-serve all-natural tomato soup (two 15-ounce cans)

Cannellini beans, drained and rinsed (half a $15\frac{1}{2}$-ounce can)

Parmesan cheese (a few tablespoons)

QUICK FIX:

Bring a medium saucepan of water to a boil. Add the pasta and cook according to package directions. A few minutes before it's done, toss in the vegetables. Bring the water back to a boil and cook until the pasta and vegetables are cooked to your liking. Drain and return to the pan. Stir in the soup and beans and heat through. Serve with Parmesan cheese.

Broths: You'll find chicken broth and vegetable broth in dozens of our recipes. Therefore, we're very picky about the products we use. When we set out to create the recipes for our book, we initially experimented with some of the low-sodium broth products on the market. Unfortunately, they were a big disappointment. Some contained monosodium glutamate (MSG), and none had the deep, rich flavor we were looking for. Next, we ruled out the regular broth and bouillon cube offerings, because most were ridiculously high in sodium (some had 1,200 milligrams per cup) and many also contained MSG. Thankfully, we were able to find two all-natural broth products that we really loved. Both had the full-bodied flavor we were looking for with under 600 milligrams of sodium in a cup. We use *Imagine Natural Organic Free Range Chicken Broth* and *Pacific Organic Free Range Chicken Broth* (packaged in shelf-stable aseptic cartons). Look for them in the health food section of your supermarket.

Tip: Once opened, all-natural broths will last seven to ten days in the refrigerator. Leftovers can also be stored in the freezer in resealable plastic bags or containers.

TOMATO PRODUCTS

A purist might cringe at the thought of using pasta sauce from a jar. But on busy weeknights, it's a compromise we're willing to make. Cooked tomato products are rich in vitamins as well as cancer-fighting antioxidants such as lycopene. The sodium content of cooked tomato products varies dramatically from product to product, so read the labels and choose wisely.

Pasta Sauce: Pasta sauce comes in just about every flavor you can imagine . . . from marinara to tomato basil to traditional. Look for a brand with less than 500 milligrams of sodium in ½ cup. We use *Classico Tomato & Basil* and *Four Cheese, Light Ragu Tomato & Basil,* and *Bertolli Tomato & Basil.*

Crushed and Diced Tomatoes: Crushed and diced tomatoes have anywhere from 80 to over 1,200 milligrams of sodium in a single cup, so check those labels.

Eat Your Lycopene

Studies suggest that eating a diet rich in the antioxidant lycopene may protect against heart disease as well as lower the risk of prostate cancer. Cooked tomato products—pasta sauce, crushed tomatoes, tomato soup, tomato juice, and ketchup—are all excellent sources. Although fresh tomatoes contain lycopene too, cooked tomato products are an even better source. Other foods with lycopene include pink grapefruit, papaya, apricots, watermelon, and guava.

PASTA, RICE, AND GRAINS

It's not a huge leap for a lot of families to switch from white bread to 100% whole wheat or whole grain, because today there are plenty of brands to choose from. In fact, some are even so soft and squishy that kids find them irresistible. But when it comes to giving your family things like whole wheat pasta and brown rice, it may be a tougher sell. Let's face it, both have a reputation for being chewy and way too "healthy" tasting. Whole grain food products, however, have come a long way since we were kids, so it's possible to stock your pantry with a healthy variety that your family won't reject.

Dried Pasta: We use many different fun-shaped pastas in our recipes to add interest . . . bow ties, shells, elbows, rotini, orzo, cavatappi, spaghetti, ziti, and no-boil lasagna noodles. In addition to your regular pastas, look for whole wheat and whole wheat blend varieties since both are higher in fiber. In our opinion, whole wheat pasta works better in some recipes than others. For example, when we tried whole wheat elbows in our Fast-As-Boxed Macaroni & Cheese (page 172), our children took one bite and said, "No way." However, whole wheat pasta works wonders in our Mini Meatballs with Whole Wheat Spaghetti (page 232) and our Sweet & Nutty Thai Thing (page 178).

Rice: Brown rice has twice as much fiber as white rice but it takes almost twice as long to cook. A simple solution is to turn to instant brown rice. By itself, instant brown rice can be a bit on the dry side, but when you mix it in with something or smother it with a sauce, it works quite well. Try it in our Shrimp Curry in a Hurry (page 260) and our One-Pot Rice & Beans (page 197). Brown rice isn't ideal for all recipes, so we also stock our pantry with flavorful jasmine rice (try it in our Sweet & Slightly Sour Shrimp, page 262). We use *Uncle Ben's* instant brown rice.

Bread: Use 100% whole wheat and whole grain breads with 2 or more grams of fiber per slice. Also, look for whole wheat pita bread, English muffins, sub rolls, and hamburger buns.

Bread Crumbs: We typically choose plain and seasoned bread crumbs made without hydrogenated oils. Don't sweat it if your brand contains hydrogenated oil, because the amount is probably negligible. Something else we like to do is make our bread crumbs from scratch by taking a stale chunk of French bread and grating it in a food processor or on a box grater.

Pizza Crust: If you've ever tried to roll out fresh pizza dough on a busy weeknight, you'll appreciate the convenience of a premade pizza crust. Perhaps the most popular brand on the market right now is Boboli, which is why we use it in some of our pizza recipes. While Boboli does in fact contain some trans fats (less than a gram per serving), we don't think it's anywhere near enough to blacklist it. If you live near a Trader Joe's, check out their pizza crust, made without any hydrogenated oils.

Tortillas and Taco Shells: When choosing a flour tortilla, look for the product with the most fiber and the least amount of fat, since the type of fat used is often hydrogenated oil or lard. Taco shells are often made with hydrogenated oil, so be on the lookout for our favorite brand. We use *Bearitos* taco shells.

Breakfast Cereal: There are literally hundreds of breakfast cereals to choose from in the supermarket. As a general rule, we buy whole grain cereals with no added sugar and at least 2 grams of fiber per serving. Some kid favorites include Wheat Chex, Raisin Bran, oatmeal, and Cheerios (also great for snacks). But breakfast cereals aren't just for breakfast. We use corn flakes as a crunchy coating for our Flaky Fish Sticks (page 248) and Rice Krispies for coating our Krispy Honey-Fried Drumsticks (page 275).

Wrap & Roll

Give us a flour tortilla and we'll give you dinner. Just about anything can be rolled up in a wrap or tortilla. Wraps are perfect when you want something fun for dinner but all you have is 5 or 10 minutes. Feel free to take our ideas and change them to suit your family's food likes and dislikes. For example, you can take our Egg & Bell Pepper Wraps and substitute diced cooked asparagus, sliced mushrooms, or chopped cooked broccoli for the peppers.

Ballpark Wraps

PANTRY ITEMS NEEDED:

> Nitrite-free hot dogs
>
> Fat-free refried beans
>
> Preshredded reduced-fat Cheddar cheese
>
> 6-inch flour tortillas
>
> Ketchup

WRAP IT UP:

Cook nitrite-free hot dogs according to package directions. While they're cooking, spread 2 to 3 tablespoons of beans and sprinkle 2 tablespoons of cheese over each tortilla. Zap them individually in the microwave for about 30 seconds, until the cheese melts and the beans are heated through. Place a cooked hot dog down the center of each tortilla, roll it up, and serve. It's the next best thing to pigs-in-a-blanket. Dip in ketchup for extra flavor. (Tip: Freeze leftover refried beans in resealable plastic bags for later use).

Cheesy Spinach Wraps

PANTRY ITEMS NEEDED:

8-inch whole wheat flour tortillas

Preshredded reduced-fat Cheddar cheese

Prewashed baby spinach

Caesar or Italian salad dressing

Roasted, shelled sunflower seeds

WRAP IT UP:

Place a tortilla on a microwave-safe plate. Arrange ¼ cup cheese, a handful of spinach leaves (½ to ¾ cup), 1 teaspoon of salad dressing, and a sprinkling of sunflower seeds over the tortilla. Heat in the microwave for 45 to 60 seconds, until the cheese melts and the spinach wilts. Roll up, cut in half, and serve.

Egg & Bell Pepper Wraps

PANTRY ITEMS NEEDED:

Olive oil

Frozen mixed pepper strips

Eggs

Preshredded reduced-fat Cheddar cheese

8-inch whole wheat flour tortillas

WRAP IT UP:

Over medium-high heat, sauté the peppers (about ½ cup per person) in a teaspoon or two of olive oil for 4 to 5 minutes. Add 1 beaten egg and 2 tablespoons of cheese per wrap and scramble for 1 to 2 minutes. Heat the tortillas in the microwave according to package directions. Arrange the egg mixture down the center, roll up, and serve.

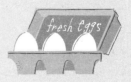

Flustered Over Flax?

Flaxseed oil, flaxseed, and flaxmeal (ground flaxseed) are rich in alpha-linolenic acid (omega-3 fats). You'll find these health-promoting items at the health food store or in the health food section of the supermarket. While the oil tends to have a sharp, unpleasant flavor, the seed and meal are easier to add to the diet. The seed, however, needs to be ground first to reap the health benefits (whole seed passes through the body undigested). Since we don't have the time or inclination to grind our own flaxseed, we simply buy the flaxmeal and add a tablespoon or two to our muffin, pancake, waffle, and cake batters. We also add it to yogurt and smoothies, and sprinkle some on our breakfast cereal. Keep in mind that flax products are perishable and should be stored in the refrigerator.

Bulgur: Bulgur is made from whole wheat kernels that have been steamed, dried, and crushed. It has a nutty flavor, a nice chewy texture, and cooks in just about 20 minutes. It's a must-have in our Bulgur & Carrot Pilaf (page 312). If you can't find bulgur in your local supermarket, ask the manager to stock it.

Couscous: Also known as Moroccan pasta, couscous is a mild-flavored grain with 2 grams of fiber per cup. We especially like the heartier-flavored whole wheat couscous with triple the fiber.

BAKING ESSENTIALS

Just because you're a Meal Makeover Mom doesn't mean you can't bake your favorite cookies, cakes, and pies. When we bake, we think, "How can we sneak some super nutrition in while we're at it?" Some of our pantry staples are designed to do just that.

Whole Wheat and All-Purpose Flour: A cup of all-purpose flour has 2 grams of fiber while 1 cup of whole wheat has 10. With five times the fiber, whole wheat is an excellent addition to baked goods. We often replace up to half of the all-purpose flour in a recipe with whole wheat. We use *King Arthur* flour.

Wheat Germ: Wheat germ has a reputation for being very healthy (and it is), but most people don't really know what to do with it. As a result, it sits on the pantry shelf unopened for years. Wheat germ is an excellent source of heart-healthy vitamin E, fiber, and folate. It's a great nutrition booster and easy to add to your recipes. When you bake muffins, pancakes, or breads, replace up to $^1/_2$ cup of all-purpose flour with $^1/_2$ cup of wheat germ. You can also sprinkle it over hot cereal or yogurt. We use wheat germ in recipes like our Brownie Mix Makeover (page 332), Banana Chocolate Chip Muffins (page 340), and Hearty Cornmeal Apple Pancakes (page 154).

Tip: Store wheat germ in the refrigerator once opened.

Cake and Brownie Mixes: If you're looking for a cake or brownie mix made without hydrogenated oils, it might take a bit of sleuthing or a trip to a natural foods supermarket. Many popular brands contain a small amount of trans fats as well as artificial colors and flavors. While you don't need to lose sleep over using mainstream mixes on occasion, it's nice to know that other great-tasting all-natural brands are also available. We use *No Pudge! Fudge Brownie Mix* and *Dr. Oetker Simple Organics Cake Mix*.

Unflavored Gelatin: Keep a box on hand to create our Better-Than-Store-Bought "Jell-O" (page 342) without the additives and artificial colors found in many prepackaged brands.

Vanilla Extract: Spend a few extra pennies and buy a good-quality, pure extract. Imitation extracts don't taste nearly as good.

Chocolate Chips: We use mini chocolate chips in some of our cookie, muffin, and dessert recipes so everyone gets a little bit of chocolate in every bite.

Pure Maple Syrup: Imitation syrup is made with corn syrup and water but little or no actual maple syrup. Go for the real thing instead.

HERBS AND SPICES

Dried seasonings can add a big kick to your cooking. Stock your pantry with the following: basil, oregano, Italian seasoning, rosemary, thyme, dill, tarragon, cloves, nutmeg, ground cinnamon, ground ginger, curry powder, chili powder, ground cumin, onion powder, and garlic powder. The

The Scoop on Kosher Salt

Some of the hottest restaurant chefs across the country use kosher salt because they think it tastes better than table salt . . . and we agree. As an added bonus, kosher salt has less sodium than regular table salt. Kosher salt is additive free and coarse in texture. Contrary to common belief, a rabbi does not "bless" the salt to make it kosher, though religious Jews do indeed use it to make meats kosher. Most of our Meal Makeover Recipes call for table salt because that's what most moms have on hand, but we suggest you stock your pantry with kosher salt as well. We also encourage you to substitute kosher salt for table salt in any of our recipes (with the exception of baked goods). We use *Diamond Crystal Kosher Salt.*

Reduced-Fat Peanut Butter: It's a Bit Nutty

	PEANUT BUTTER (PER 2 TABLESPOONS)	REDUCED-FAT PEANUT BUTTER (PER 2 TABLESPOONS)	ALL-NATURAL PEANUT BUTTER (PER 2 TABLESPOONS)
Calories	190	190	200
Total Fat (g)	17	12	16
Saturated Fat (g)	3.5	2.5	2
Carbohydrate (g)	7	15	7
Sugar (g)	3	5	2
Protein (g)	7	7	7
Fiber (g)	2	2	2
Ingredients	Roasted peanuts, sugar, partially hydrogenated vegetable oils, salt	Roasted peanuts, corn syrup solids, sugar, soy protein, salt, partially hydrogenated vegetable oils, mono- and diglycerides	Peanuts, salt

shelf life of herbs and spices is anywhere from 1 to 3 years. While they won't spoil, they can lose their flavor. When substituting with fresh herbs, use about 1 tablespoon of fresh for every 1 teaspoon of dried.

Nuts, Seeds, and Dried Fruit

Using nuts as a topping for fish, adding sunflower seeds to a quiche, and blending golden raisins into a savory coleslaw are simple ways to kick up the flavor and good nutrition of a dish.

Nuts: Walnuts, pecans, pine nuts, cashews, almonds, and peanuts (technically a legume, not a nut) get a bad rap because they contain fat. But bear in mind that most of that fat is the healthy kind. Nuts are also packed with vitamins, minerals, and antioxidants . . . so enjoy a handful here and there and use them in recipes like Walnut-Crusted Salmon (page 258), Olive Oil's Orzo (page 310), and Our Favorite Chocolate Cookie (page 324). Nuts are best stored in the refrigerator or freezer. If someone in your family has an allergy to peanuts or tree nuts, just leave them out of the recipe.

Peanut Butter: What could be easier and healthier than a peanut butter and jelly sandwich? Peanut butter is an inexpensive source of protein and heart-healthy monounsaturated fats. Some kids like it smooth, while others prefer it chunky. What we like are the all-natural brands, because all they contain are peanuts and salt. If you're wondering whether the reduced-fat varieties are worth a try, consider that, ironically, they often contain the same number of calories as the regular version, but less of the good fats. We don't see the point of replacing some of the good fat with sugar. We use *Smuckers Natural Peanut Butter, Trader Joe's Peanut Butter,* and *Teddy Old Fashioned Peanut Butter.*

Sunflower Seeds: Sunflower seeds are a good source of healthy fats, fiber, and vitamin E, an antioxidant that protects the heart. Use them for homemade trail mixes, in recipes like our Sunny Broccoli Slaw (page 319), or sprinkle them over salads.

Dried Fruit: Raisins and dried plums (aka prunes) add sweetness, flavor, and fiber to a dish, not to mention a host of disease-fighting antioxidants. Go "out of the box" and try dried plums in our Beef & Sweet Potato Stew (page 236) or raisins in our Moroccan Un-Stuffed Peppers (page 284).

The Meal Makeover Moms' Refrigerator

Have you ever found a UFO (unidentified funky object) in your refrigerator? You know, the squishy, rotten cucumber or the green moldy lemon hiding in the back of your vegetable bin. Your refrigerator can get just as cluttered and disorganized as your cupboards, making daily dinner preparation more of a challenge than it needs to be.

We suggest you set aside a few minutes each week to take stock of what is or is not in your refrigerator. A good time to do this is right before you go grocery shopping or when you're planning your meals for the week. While you're getting organized, be sure to move last week's yogurts, sour cream, milk, and other perishable items to the front of your fridge so your family eats those first, before the newer ones. A good way to remember this rule is "FIFO" (first in, first out). Also take a moment to monitor the temperature of your refrigerator. If you don't have a refrigerator thermometer, you can buy one for under ten dollars. To keep bacteria from having a picnic in your fridge, keep the temperature between 34 and 40 degrees F.

DAIRY

Dairy foods are a great source of bone-building calcium, and they're perhaps one of the easiest foods to get into your family's diet. Today, a variety of great-tasting, reduced-fat dairy foods makes it possible to get your calcium without going overboard on saturated fat and calories.

1% Lowfat Milk: An 8-ounce glass of 1% milk has 1.5 grams of saturated fat versus 5 grams in a cup of whole milk. Another bonus: The amount of calcium in lowfat milk is actually a bit higher than in whole. If your family prefers soymilk, choose a product that's fortified with calcium and vitamin D.

Preshredded Reduced-Fat Cheese: To save time in the kitchen, stock your fridge with preshredded cheese instead of shredding it yourself from a block. Shaving 5 minutes from your prep time can really take the sting out of having to make dinner *again*. You'll appreciate this shortcut ingredient the next time you make one of our pizzas or our Fast-As-Boxed Macaroni & Cheese (page 172). Choose reduced-fat Cheddar, Mexican blend, and part-skim mozzarella cheese.

Parmesan Cheese: Parmesan cheese is one of our favorite flavor enhancers. If available, choose the more flavorful fresh grated Parmesan.

Butter: Some recipes just wouldn't be the same without it. Although butter contains saturated fat, a little bit goes a long way. Just make our Corn & Carrot Chowder (page 108), and you'll see what we mean. Given the choice between butter and margarine, we'd opt for butter most of the time. Besides the fact that the taste of butter can't be beat, many margarine products are made with hydrogenated oils and therefore contain unhealthy trans fats. If you do use margarine, look for a product that is trans fat free.

Reduced-Fat Sour Cream: Sour cream can have 15 to 20 grams of saturated fat in $1/2$ cup. Switch to reduced-fat and you'll shave more than half without losing the real sour cream flavor. The reason we don't use fat-free sour cream in our recipes is because it just doesn't taste as good as the reduced-fat stuff.

Yogurt: To give your family a meal makeover, there is no reason to shop for low-calorie, fat-free yogurts made with artificial sweeteners. Yuck! There are plenty of other delicious, "real"-tasting options to choose from. We like to keep a large carton of vanilla yogurt on hand for after-school snacks (mix with some granola or fruit) and for using in our Chocolate Pudding with Toppers (page 322). We use *Stonyfield Farm Yogurt* and *Yoplait*.

Omega-3 Eggs: Every time we break an egg, we feel good about it. Not only are eggs a superb source of high-quality protein, certain brands contain healthy omega-3 fatty acids as well (the kind of fat found in some seafood). Omega-3 eggs come from hens fed a diet of algae, fish oil, or flaxseed. In general, eggs stay fresh for 1 month in the refrigerator. We use *Gold Circle Farms* and *Egg-Lands Best* (check your supermarket for other regional brands).

PRODUCE

While some folks might consider Fruit Roll Ups and French fries members of the fruit and vegetable family, we favor carrots, spinach, bell peppers, strawberries, and other nutrient-packed produce instead. Rich in vitamins, minerals, and fiber as well as antioxidants such as lutein (vital for eye health) and beta-carotene (protective against heart disease and certain cancers), experts tell us to eat at least 5 servings of fruits and vegetables a day. When possible, shop for organic and locally grown produce.

Fruit: Did you know that refrigerated apples last up to ten times longer than apples left at room temperature? Did you know the world's most popular fruit is the tomato followed by bananas, apples, oranges, and watermelon? And did you know that pears, peaches, plums, tomatoes, and bananas ripen faster when they're placed in a sealed brown paper bag? It's hard to go overboard on fresh fruit. Keep a wide variety on hand and try new things from time to time, including mangoes, kiwis, fresh pineapple, cantaloupe, and cherries (watch out for those pits!).

Vegetables: If you're too busy to slice and dice your vegetables, just stroll down the produce aisle and look for ready-to-eat baby carrots, coleslaw mix, broccoli slaw mix, prewashed baby spinach, presliced mushrooms, scallop-cut potatoes, and more. The refrigerated section of the produce aisle is a Meal Makeover Mom's delight.

Tip: Always keep a bag of large carrots in your fridge. In just one minute flat, you can peel and shred a carrot and then add it to your sandwich, soup, and casserole recipes. Try it in our Carrot-Top Tuna (page 125), Mama's Amazing Ziti (page 174), and Hungry Kids Goulash (page 238).

Olives: From mild canned olives to the more intensely flavored kalamatas, use them in recipes for extra flavor and monounsaturated fats.

Lemon Juice and Lime Juice: Come on . . . admit it. We know you probably have one of those cute little plastic lemons or limes in your fridge right now (there are support groups for people like you!). Guess what? You'll find them in our refrigerators, too. Bottled lemon juice and lime juice come in handy whenever a recipe calls for a tablespoon or two and the fresh ones are nowhere to be found in your fridge.

100% Fruit Juices: Orange juice and apple juice aren't just for drinking with meals and snacks. They also work well when used in some of our recipes. Avoid juice drinks made with added sugar and choose calcium-fortified juices if your family doesn't get enough calcium elsewhere.

Garlic and Ginger: Fresh garlic and ginger add kick to whatever you're cooking. For added convenience, turn to bottled, crushed, or minced garlic and ginger.

Meat, Poultry, and Seafood

If your family eats one or two seafood dishes a week, you're well on your way to a healthy meal makeover. Seafood, especially salmon, is a rich source of healthy omega-3 fats. Seafood is also an excellent source of protein, as is beef, pork, and chicken. Go for the leanest cuts of pork and beef you can find (for the leanest cuts, see page 243) and shop for skinless chicken to keep saturated fat in check.

Deli Meats and Hot Dogs

No matter how you slice them, deli meats can be very high in fat and sodium. Many also contain nitrites. Look for lean, lower-sodium deli meats and, if you can find them, those made without nitrites. As for hot dogs, most contain nitrites too, so shop for vegetarian hot dogs or all-natural, nitrite-free varieties (see Best of the Bunch, page 55). We use *Coleman All Natural Uncured Beef Hot Dogs, Hans' All Natural Uncured Beef Hot Dogs,* and *Applegate Farms Beef Hot Dogs.*

Tofu

If you or someone in your family is a vegetarian, you probably cook with tofu already. But for most of the carnivores out there, tofu is a mystery. We believe it's time to give tofu a chance. That's why we use it in our Tasty Tofu Nuggets (page 206) and Mixed-Up Tofu (page 204). You can also cook it up on the grill. All you have to do is cut a block of tofu into eight or nine slices, drain between paper towels, and then marinate for about 30 minutes in a mixture of honey and lite teriyaki sauce or honey and Thai peanut sauce. Cook about 3 minutes per side on your grill and enjoy.

The Meal Makeover Moms' Freezer

Sometimes we wish that our freezers were bigger than our refrigerators. That's because a surprising number of the foods we rely on for healthy, everyday cooking come from the frozen food aisle. Take frozen vegetables, for example. While we certainly love fresh vegetables, on crazy nights when we don't have the time to wash, chop, and cook them, a bag of frozen mixed vegetables or a box of frozen chopped broccoli can sure come in handy.

It's important to keep tabs on the contents of not only your refrigerator and kitchen cupboards, but also your freezer. After all, you can only keep foods in your freezer for so long before the dreaded freezer burn sets in. According to experts at the FDA, freezer burn happens when air reaches the surface of your food and dries it out. Freezer burn isn't a food safety issue but it *is* a food quality issue since it can ruin the flavor of your food. To stop freezer burn in its tracks, keep your freezer at or below o degrees F, wrap your food tightly in plastic wrap or aluminum foil (or store in an airtight container), and monitor how long foods have been in your freezer. Your best bet is to store ground beef no longer than 3 to 4 months, steak 6 to 12 months, poultry 10 months, hot dogs 1 to 2 months, and frozen veggies up to 8 months.

A final word on freezers: Since freezing does *not* destroy harmful bacteria, avoid thawing frozen foods on your kitchen counter. At room temperature, bacteria can grow and multiply. The best way to thaw frozen foods is in the refrigerator. You can also thaw in the microwave oven or place the sealed food item in a bowl of cold water, changing the water every 30 minutes.

PRODUCE

Never rule out frozen produce, because it can actually be nutritionally superior to fresh. When fruits and vegetables are processed immediately after harvest (when the nutrients are at their peak), they retain more of their vitamins, minerals, and phytonutrients as compared to produce that may have sat on a truck for a week or more before reaching your store. Worth noting too are all the new organic frozen fruits and vegetables now available in most supermarkets.

Vegetables: Besides the old standbys of corn kernels, peas, carrots, mixed veggies, spinach, cauliflower, and potatoes, the freezer section is now brimming with new-and-improved choices. Look for frozen kale (a great addition to our Mashed Potatoes with Kale (really!), page 306), hash brown potatoes, mixed bell peppers, collard greens, stir-fry mixes, and broccoli florets (if you've ever given your kids those big, soggy spears, you'll appreciate the appeal of florets).

Fruits: Frozen blueberries, strawberries, raspberries, mangoes, and even peaches work wonders in fruit smoothies as well as in homemade desserts. Use frozen blueberries for our delicious Blueberry Snack Cake (page 330).

PASTA

For a last-minute meal that kids are sure to devour, turn to frozen tortellini and ravioli. Toss them with pasta sauce, a drizzle of extra virgin olive oil and Parmesan cheese, or get adventurous and try our Tortellini with Broccoli "Pesto" (page 180) or our Cheese Ravioli with Pumpkin Sauce (page 176).

MEAT AND SEAFOOD

When lean cuts of beef, pork, or skinless, boneless chicken breast are on sale, buy an extra pound or two and freeze them for later use. Remember to wrap them tight to avoid freezer burn. Also keep frozen precooked shrimp and lowfat breakfast sausage on hand to liven up your usual dinner repertoire. Check out our Shrimp "Not-So-Fried" Rice (page 264) and our Super Sausage & Broccoli Strata (page 166). We use *Jones Light Sausage & Rice Links*.

MEAT-FREE GROUNDS

If you've ever walked by frozen meat-free "grounds" in the supermarket, you may have wondered what they're for. Meat-free grounds are typically made from soy. Another frozen product, called Quorn, is made from a mushroomlike derivative (it sounds unusual, but it's really quite good!). They're ideal for casseroles. We use *Quorn* in our Easy Enchilada Casserole (page 202).

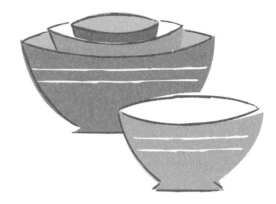

Pantry Maintenance

It's hard to maintain a well-stocked pantry without a well-organized shopping list. Of course, your shopping list may not look exactly like your neighbors', because after all, everyone's food likes, dislikes, and favorite recipes vary. If you're used to writing your shopping list on a scrap of paper, you'll love our Meal Makeover Moms' Shopping List, organized aisle by aisle. Go to our web site, www.mealmakeovermoms.com, and customize your own or create one based on our sample below.

MEAL MAKEOVER MOMS' SHOPPING LIST

PRODUCE AISLE

- ☐ Apples
- ☐ Avocado
- ☐ Bananas
- ☐ Berries
- ☐ Cantaloupe
- ☐ Grapes
- ☐ Mangoes
- ☐ Oranges
- ☐ Pears
- ☐ Asparagus
- ☐ Bell peppers
- ☐ Broccoli
- ☐ Broccoli slaw
- ☐ Carrots, baby
- ☐ Carrots, large
- ☐ Carrots, preshredded
- ☐ Coleslaw mix
- ☐ Eggplant
- ☐ Lettuce, Romaine
- ☐ Mushrooms, presliced
- ☐ Potatoes, scalloped
- ☐ Spinach, prewashed baby
- ☐ Sweet potatoes
- ☐ Tomatoes
- ☐ Tomatoes, grape
- ☐ Zucchini
- ☐ _____
- ☐ _____
- ☐ _____

FROZEN FOOD AISLE

- ☐ Blueberries
- ☐ Raspberries
- ☐ Strawberries
- ☐ Bell peppers, mixed
- ☐ Broccoli florets
- ☐ Carrots
- ☐ Cauliflower
- ☐ Collard greens
- ☐ Corn kernels
- ☐ Kale
- ☐ Lima beans, baby
- ☐ Peas
- ☐ Potatoes, hash brown
- ☐ Spinach
- ☐ Vegetables, mixed
- ☐ Ravioli
- ☐ Tortellini
- ☐ Sausage, lowfat breakfast
- ☐ Shrimp, cooked
- ☐ _____
- ☐ _____
- ☐ _____
- ☐ _____

DAIRY AISLE

- ☐ Butter
- ☐ Cheddar cheese, preshredded reduced-fat
- ☐ Cottage cheese, 1% lowfat
- ☐ Cream cheese, light
- ☐ Eggs, omega-3
- ☐ Feta cheese
- ☐ Milk, 1% lowfat
- ☐ Mozzarella cheese, preshredded part-skim
- ☐ Orange juice w/calcium
- ☐ Parmesan cheese, grated
- ☐ Ricotta cheese, part-skim
- ☐ Sour cream, reduced-fat
- ☐ Yogurt, lowfat fruit
- ☐ Yogurt, lowfat vanilla
- ☐ _____
- ☐ _____
- ☐ _____

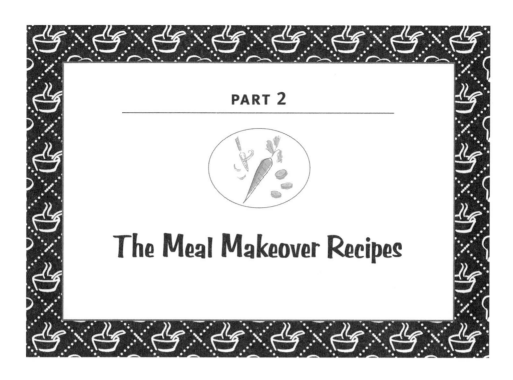

PART 2

The Meal Makeover Recipes

There are literally millions of recipes out there—in cookbooks, on the Internet, in magazines and newspapers, and in Grandma's old recipe box. The challenge is in finding a recipe that "has it all": one that is nutrient packed but still tastes great, appeals to the entire family, is easy to make, and can be on the table in minutes not hours. That can be a tall order . . . but that's exactly what you'll find in the second part of our book. For those moms who've been taking the path of least resistance—eating out, ordering pizza, and relying on frozen and boxed meals to feed their families—we're here to say there are plenty of other options.

Because we understand your daily dinnertime dilemma, we decided to take some of the most popular family favorites, things like spaghetti & meatballs, lasagna, fried chicken, macaroni & cheese, mashed potatoes, and chocolate chip cookies, and give them a makeover. Our criteria were simple: to sneak super nutrition into each recipe . . . making it healthier than the original, maintaining or improving the flavor, and speeding up the prep and cook time whenever possible. In order to do that, we:

🥕 Added vegetables and fruit to increase the vitamins, minerals, phytonutrients (plant nutrients), and fiber.

🥕 Used whole grains to increase the nutrients and fiber.

❤ Switched to lowfat dairy and lean meats to lower the saturated fat and calories.

❤ Chose convenience foods wisely to provide desperately needed shortcuts in the kitchen while limiting the addition of trans fats and sodium.

❤ Replaced much of the butter, margarine, and shortening with healthier oils such as canola oil and olive oil to reduce the saturated fat and trans fats.

❤ Kept a watchful eye on portion sizes to keep the calories in check.

The results of our efforts are 120 fast and easy weeknight recipes that provide many of the nutrients that may otherwise be lacking or missing from your family's diet. For example, in our makeover for bean burritos, we add a sweet potato (an unlikely but delicious ingredient), bursting with beta-carotene and other health-enhancing nutrients. Spaghetti & meatballs also gets kicked up a few nutritional notches when we switch to lean ground beef and use whole wheat spaghetti in order to slash the saturated fat and triple the fiber. If you are looking for fat-free recipes, you won't find them here because fat makes food taste good. Certain fats, namely monounsaturated and polyunsaturated fats, found in such things as olive oil, canola oil, nuts, and avocados, are also vital to good health, so we use them without guilt! Even if you're watching your weight, research shows that a moderate amount of fat can make a lower-calorie diet more palatable and easier to follow over the long haul.

We spent countless hours in our kitchens developing, testing, and retesting each and every recipe. We even had moms like you try them out to make sure their families loved them as much as ours did. In reality, however, we don't expect that you and your family will be wowed by all 120 recipes. After all, every person within a family has different food likes and dislikes (and as you know, some of those preferences can change with the wind), making it a challenge to feed the family every night. Our recipes simply give you more choices, more options, and more ideas, because we know that the meals moms make over and over again can get a bit tiresome after a while. If you can find even a few recipes in each chapter to add to your existing recipe repertoire, we consider that a huge success.

As Meal Makeover Moms, many of you will be striving to lower the saturated fat and trans fats at your family's table, keep calories under control, and eat more fruits, vegetables, and whole grains. Our recipes help you to achieve those very goals. There is no doubt that when you prepare a nourishing meal for your family, you make a positive impact on their health. It's an exciting opportunity, so get cooking!

Meal Makeover Moms' Q & A

After creating all 120 recipes for *The Moms' Guide to Meal Makeovers,* we asked busy moms to try them out. Having "testers" all across the country was a great way to work out the kinks and clarify our directions. We asked our moms to "tell all" and to be as critical as possible. What follows are some of the cooking concerns and questions that popped up along the way.

Q: What's the best way to thaw frozen vegetables?

A: You can thaw frozen vegetables by heating them in the microwave or running them under hot water and then draining. Either way, the reason we often suggest thawing is because it speeds up the cooking time.

Q: What's the best way to steam vegetables?

A: Set a vegetable steamer in a medium saucepan with 1 to 2 inches of water. Add your vegetables to the steamer, cover, and bring to a boil. Reduce the heat and simmer until the veggies are crisp, tender, mushy, or however you like them.

Q: How should I shred a carrot?

A: Shredding a carrot takes about a minute. First, peel the carrot then shred it on the medium or large holes of a box grater or run it through a food processor. Shredded carrots cook faster than diced and blend nicely into recipes.

Q: Should I use organic fruits and vegetables?

A: Currently, American families consume too few fruits and vegetables so our number one goal right now is to encourage people to eat more of them. If you choose to feed your family organic produce grown without the use of pesticides, we fully support your efforts. Most supermarkets today stock a variety of fresh and frozen organic produce. If the price fits into your food budget, by all means, go organic!

Q: I was surprised to see corn kernels in some of your recipes. Isn't corn considered one of those nutritionally inferior vegetables?

A: As far as we're concerned, no vegetable is nutritionally inferior. Corn contains two antioxidants, lutein and zeaxanthin, which research shows may ward off cataracts and the blinding eye condition, macular degeneration.

Q: If a recipe calls for frozen or canned vegetables, can I substitute fresh?

A: Absolutely. We often use frozen and canned because most of our recipes are meant to be last-minute meals—something you can whip up when you walk in the door and there's little time to cook. By all means, feel free to substitute fresh produce for frozen or canned or vice versa. It's a personal choice. Believe it or not, sometimes frozen and canned produce can be "fresher" than fresh (if you've ever run across a limp, rubbery head of broccoli at the supermarket you'll know what we mean). If you're lucky enough to have a farmer's market in your area, we encourage you to shop there for freshly picked, locally grown produce.

Q: What's better, kosher salt or table salt? I noticed you use both in your recipes.

A: In most of our recipes we use table salt because that's what moms typically have on hand. That said, however, we prefer the taste of *Diamond Crystal Kosher Salt* and the fact that it has half as much sodium as table salt. We call for kosher salt in some of our recipes, including those for Simply Delicious Broccoli (page 318) and Finally Edible Brussels Sprouts (page 317) where it really helps to bring out the flavor of the vegetables. As a rule of thumb, you can substitute kosher salt for table salt anytime (with the exception of baking, where exact amounts are critical).

Q: Some of your recipes call for nuts. What do I do if my child is allergic?

A: Indeed, we use nuts from time to time to enhance the nutritional value and flavor of our recipes. If your child has a nut allergy, leave the nuts out, or move on to one of our other delicious, kid-friendly recipes.

Q: What's the best way to toast walnuts, pecans, and other nuts?

A: We use one of two methods to toast nuts. For method number one, place the nuts in a single layer on a baking sheet and bake at 325°F in the oven or toaster oven until golden brown, about 6 minutes. Stir the nuts or shake the baking sheet occasionally to ensure even baking. For the second method, place the nuts in a dry skillet over medium heat. Cook, stirring frequently, until golden brown, about 5 minutes. Toasting brings out the flavor and aroma . . . just keep a watchful eye, because nuts can burn easily.

Q: How should I chop nuts?

A: To chop nuts, place them on a cutting board and chop with a sharp chef's knife, or place in a food processor and pulse a few turns (be careful not to overprocess, otherwise you'll end up with paste). Finely and very finely chopped nuts should be similar in size to coarse sea salt, while coarsely chopped nuts should be a bit larger, about the size of small dried lentils.

Q: When I make pasta, I usually cook the entire box for my family of four. Is that too much pasta?

A: In a word . . . yes! Pasta is sometimes perceived as "fattening" because people simply eat too much of it—and eating too much of anything can pack on the pounds. In our recipes, we typically call for 2 ounces of dried pasta per person (that's about 1 cup cooked). Watching the pasta portion size leaves ample room for other nourishing foods, such as fruits, vegetables, and lean meats and dairy.

Q: What are thin-sliced chicken cutlets and what should I do if I can't find them?

A: Thin-sliced chicken cutlets can be found in the same supermarket section as other fresh poultry products. Even though the cutlets are a bit more expensive, we use them because they are trimmed of all the fat, easy to work with, and cook up in a matter of minutes . . . saving valuable time in the kitchen. If you can't find the thin-sliced chicken cutlets, make your own by placing skinless, boneless chicken breast halves between two sheets of plastic wrap or wax paper. Using a meat mallet or the bottom of a small saucepan, flatten to ¼-inch thickness.

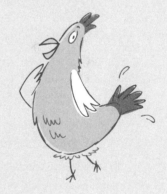

Q: In several of your soup recipes and those that include a cheese sauce, you tell us to whisk flour together with milk. What's the purpose of this?

A: Soups and sauces can be thickened without the use of heavy cream and butter. To do this, we use our Slurry in a Hurry. See our sidebar on page 107 for details.

Recipe Format: What to Expect

Our recipes are chock-full of information. As you read them, here's what you'll find:

SERVINGS

It's hard to determine how many people a recipe will feed when some families have two toddlers while others have two teens. Since we don't know the age or size of your family, we decided to base our suggested servings for each recipe on young families such as our own. Janice has a three- and a ten-year-old, while Liz has a four- and a seven-year-old. Clearly, if you have two teenage boys at home, you may need to make some adjustments to our recipes, such as adding more chicken here or a cup of pasta there. But if you have two small children, you may have leftovers.

"QUICK PREP" SYMBOL

A clock symbol 🕐 🕐 appearing at the top of a recipe signifies that the recipe is particularly fast and easy and can be on the table in 15 or 30 minutes.

RECIPE INTRODUCTION

Most of our "before" recipes came from friends and family members or from one of three popular family cookbooks. In the introduction, we describe the recipe and its nutritional shortcomings. Sometimes we toss in an amusing story or helpful hint on getting kids to try new things.

MOMS MAKE IT OVER BY . . .

This section explains how we gave the "before" recipe a face-lift. We might tell you that we added carrots for vitamins, minerals, phytonutrients, and fiber or that we lowered the saturated fat by replacing a stick of butter with a few tablespoons of healthy olive oil. It's a real eye-opener! We promise not to bog you down with too much science here, so we won't be listing all umpteen hundred nutrients in each ingredient.

INGREDIENTS

Our ingredients are simple and straightforward. While we often rely on convenience foods like pasta sauce, frozen veggies, and all-natural chicken broth to get you to the table quickly, we shy away from most things made with partially hydrogenated vegetable oils and shortening. In general, we also avoid foods with monosodium glutamate (for The Trouble with MSG, see page 74), excessive amounts of saturated fat and sodium, and artificial colors and flavors. Refer back to our pantry chapter (page 70) for specific product guidance and suggestions. If we happen to call for an ingredient you think your family will reject, then by all means leave it out or substitute something else for it. The same holds true for the degree to which you season your food. If your family loves fiery flavors, feel free to increase the amount of spices or use things like hot salsa versus mild. It's your choice.

DIRECTIONS

We made our directions as clear and concise as humanly possible yet certain things may still confuse you. That's why we wrote the *Makeover Moms' Q & A* that follows. After reading it, if there is anything you still don't understand, please visit our web site, www.mealmakeovermoms.com, and send us an e-mail with your questions. The last thing we would ever want is for you to stress out over recipe directions during the dinner hour.

MOMS' KITCHEN NOTES

Here, we offer serving suggestions, fun facts, substitution ideas, and additional information about each recipe.

NUTRITION INFORMATION

All recipes were analyzed using the Food Processor nutrition analysis software by ESHA Research. We included information on calories, total fat, saturated fat, sodium, carbohydrate, fiber, and protein. The BEFORE column lists the nutrient breakdown for the original recipe while the AFTER column reflects our made-over version. If a recipe serves 6 to 8, we use 7 for our analysis. Optional ingredients are not included in the analysis.

Bear in mind that the numbers, while impressive, don't always tell the entire story. Adding things like fruits, vegetables, whole grains, beans, and nuts to a recipe (which is what we're all about) enhances the health benefits well beyond what the nutritional numbers could ever reflect. Also keep in mind that from time to time, our makeover recipe may have slightly more fat than the original. Don't be alarmed; rest assured, the fat in our recipes is the good kind that can improve the health of your family.

To put our numbers into even greater perspective, consider the following: In general, the average person who consumes 2,000 calories a day is advised to:

- Keep total fat intake to 65 to 75 grams per day
- Limit saturated fat to less than 20 grams per day
- Limit sodium to less than 2,400 milligrams per day
- Eat about 250 grams of carbohydrate per day

- Eat 25 to 38 grams of fiber per day
- Consume 75 to 100 grams of protein per day

Our Favorite Makeovers

We have often been asked which recipes are our personal favorites. While it's hard to choose because we obviously like them all, we came up with the following winners!

THE BISSEX FAMILY

Janice: Sweet & Nutty Thai Thing (page 178)

Don: Walnut-Crusted Salmon (page 258)

Carolyn (age 10): Mexican Lasagna (page 228)

Leah (age 3): Blueberry Banana Pancakes (page 152)

THE WEISS/CARRUTHERS FAMILY

Liz: Creamy Stroganoff with Peas (page 230)

Tim: Oh-So-Easy Chicken Parmesan (page 286)

Josh (age 7): Cheesy Broccoli Soup (page 116)

Simon (age 4): Banana Chocolate Chip Muffins (page 340)

CHAPTER 5

Souped-Up Soups & Stews

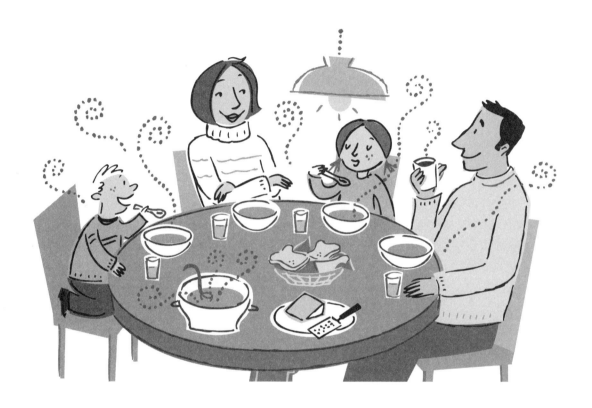

B.L.T. in a Bowl • A-Plus Alphabet Soup • Last-Minute Black Bean Soup • Corn & Carrot Chowder • Salmon Seashell Chowder • Orange Soup • Kale, Sweet Potato, & Kielbasa Soup • Shrimpy Green Coconut Soup • Cheesy Broccoli Soup • Chicken Stew with Baby Carrots • Halftime Taco Chili • White Bean Cassoulet Soup

oups and stews are the quintessential comfort food. Every mom knows that. For Liz, whose Jewish roots shine through every time one of her boys gets sick, chicken soup is a must. Janice, the sports fanatic between us, loves to host tailgate parties when football season rolls around and yes, you guessed it, hearty stews and chili are always the main attraction on her table.

At their best, soups and stews are swift, simple, and soothing, not to mention a complete source of everything you need in a meal—protein, complex carbohydrates, and healthy fats. But, they can also be way too salty and high in saturated fat. If you do make your soups and stews from scratch, keep in mind that many of the broth products and bouillon cubes on the market are astoundingly high in sodium. As for the canned soups that busy moms often fall back on when there's barely enough time to grab the can opener, well, besides the salt issue, some of them also contain monosodium glutamate (MSG), chicken fat, and partially hydrogenated vegetable oils. Our best advice is to choose wisely.

In this chapter, we highlight simple soup solutions that improve the taste and nutritional profile of a dozen old and new favorites. First, we show you how to take a basic can of soup and *soup it up* to be heartier and healthier. Our B.L.T. in a Bowl (page 103), for example, begins with 30%-less-sodium tomato soup. To that, we toss in some tortellini, fresh baby spinach, and bacon bits. All of a sudden, it's a filling, satisfying meal. Next, we lighten up old classics, slashing the salt and saturated fat while tossing in nutritious and delicious ingredients. Our A-Plus Alphabet Soup (page 105) offers an alternative to store-bought alphabet soup. Our homemade version is prepared with lots of colorful vegetables as well as protein and iron-rich chickpeas.

Last, but certainly not least, we offer easy ways to cut corners. Purchasing a high-quality, all-natural chicken broth instead of making it from scratch is an obvious shortcut strategy, but did you ever consider a bag of frozen butternut squash for butternut squash soup? We did and it worked wonders, saving time in the kitchen as well as aggravation (if you've ever tried to slice open a big, bulky butternut squash you'll know what we mean).

So whether you slurp them or savor every spoonful, soups and stews are an appetizing addition to any meal makeover.

B.L.T. in a Bowl

MAKES 4 SERVINGS

What happens when you take the basic ingredients in a B.L.T. sandwich—bacon, lettuce, and tomato—and transform them into a hearty bowl of soup? The answer: a B.L.T. in a Bowl. We created this recipe after hearing from moms who felt guilty every time they opened a can of tomato soup and called it dinner. Sure, tomato soup is a source of lycopene, an antioxidant that may ward off certain cancers, and kids certainly love it, but it's a far cry from a stick-to-your-ribs meal. Our awesome soup, made with tomato soup as the base along with spinach, tortellini, and bacon bits, proves that convenience foods can work to your nutritional advantage.

Moms Make It Over By . . .

- Adding spinach for vitamins, minerals, phytonutrients, and fiber.
- Including tortellini to make it a heartier meal.

Two 10¾-ounce cans 30%-less-sodium tomato soup

2 cans water

6 to 8 ounces frozen cheese tortellini

One 6-ounce bag prewashed baby spinach (about 4 packed cups)

4 teaspoons real bacon bits

2 tablespoons grated Parmesan cheese, optional

1. Pour the tomato soup and water into a large saucepan and stir to combine. Cover and bring to a boil.

2. Add the tortellini and cook, uncovered, according to package directions, stirring frequently. Do not drain. Stir in the spinach and cook until wilted, about 2 minutes.

3. Serve in individual bowls and top with bacon bits and Parmesan cheese as desired.

PREPARATION TIME: 5 MINUTES
COOKING TIME: 10 MINUTES

	Before	After
Calories	100	260
Fat (g)	2.5	4
Saturated Fat (g)	0	1.5
Sodium (mg)	850	780
Carbohydrate (g)	20	47
Fiber (g)	<1	3
Protein (g)	2	7

Soup It Up: Five Easy Makeovers for a Can of Soup

Store-bought soups are often high in sodium and some are also high in fat. Thankfully, food companies now offer all-natural brands as well as lighter versions of many old favorites including cream of mushroom soup, New England clam chowder, and tomato soup. While stripping some of the saturated fat and sodium from savory soups is an excellent start, it's just one step to improving your family's diet. To soup up your favorite reduced-sodium and reduced-fat canned soups, stir in extra ingredients to kick up the good nutrition. The final result will be a more satisfying, nourishing bowl.

CANNED SOUP	ADD-INS	SOUPED-UP RESULTS
1 can tomato soup	Lean deli ham, diced Frozen peas, thawed	More protein More fiber
1 can New England clam chowder	Frozen corn kernels, thawed	More nutrients such as lutein and zeaxanthin; antioxidants good for eye health More fiber
1 can cream of mushroom soup	One 8-ounce package presliced mushrooms, sautéed	More flavor More fiber
1 can chicken noodle soup	Canned cannellini beans or chickpeas, drained and rinsed	More fiber More protein
1 can creamy potato soup	Frozen baby broccoli florets, thawed	More flavor More fiber More nutrients such as vitamin C; good for chronic disease prevention

A-Plus Alphabet Soup

MAKES 4 SERVINGS

We've never met a kid who didn't love alphabet soup. Moms love it too for its simplicity. Walk in the door, open a can, and heat it up. But read the label and you may see ingredients like monosodium glutamate and not enough protein or calories to call it a meal. With the help of Janice's daughter Carolyn, we concocted our own homemade version brimming with colorful vegetables and hearty, iron-rich chickpeas. Notice how the little pasta letters grow bigger the longer they sit in the bowl.

Moms Make It Over By . . .

🍓 Adding mixed vegetables for vitamins, minerals, phytonutrients, and fiber.

🍓 Including chickpeas for added nutrients and fiber.

> 2 cups all-natural chicken broth or vegetable broth
>
> One 8-ounce can tomato sauce
>
> 4 ounces dried alphabet pasta (about ¾ cup)
>
> 1½ cups frozen mixed vegetables, thawed
>
> One 7¾-ounce can chickpeas, drained and rinsed
>
> ¼ cup grated Parmesan cheese, optional

1. Add the broth, 1½ cups water, and tomato sauce to a medium saucepan and stir to combine. Cover and bring to a boil.

2. Add the pasta, vegetables, and chickpeas, and boil gently, uncovered, until the pasta is done, 6 to 8 minutes. Stir occasionally.

3. Serve in bowls and top with Parmesan cheese as desired.

PREPARATION TIME: 5 MINUTES

COOKING TIME: 10 MINUTES

	Before	After
Calories	90	230
Fat (g)	0.5	1
Saturated Fat (g)	0	0
Sodium (mg)	860	670
Carbohydrate (g)	18	46
Fiber (g)	2	7
Protein (g)	3	10

Last-Minute Black Bean Soup

MAKES 4 SERVINGS

A lot of traditional black bean soup recipes call for dried beans. We're all for tradition, but as far as we're concerned, the thought of soaking the beans and then sitting around for hours while they simmer is worse than listening to your child practice the violin for the very first time. Our soup solution was to use canned black beans instead. They're just as nutritious as the dried kind, considerably more convenient, and an easy way to get a nourishing bowl of soup on the table in a matter of minutes.

Moms Make It Over By . . .

- Adding corn and salsa for vitamins, minerals, phytonutrients, and fiber.
- Eliminating the butter and salt pork to lower the saturated fat and calories.

> One 19-ounce can black beans, undrained
> 1½ cups frozen corn kernels
> ½ cup salsa
> 1 tablespoon bottled or fresh lime juice
> ½ to 1 teaspoon chili powder
> ½ to 1 teaspoon ground cumin
> ¼ cup preshredded reduced-fat Cheddar cheese
> ½ cup reduced-fat sour cream, optional

1. In a medium saucepan, combine the beans, corn, salsa, ½ cup water, lime juice, chili powder, and cumin. Cover and bring to a boil. Reduce the heat and simmer, uncovered, about 5 minutes.

2. Serve in individual bowls and top with the cheese and sour cream as desired.

PREPARATION TIME: 5 MINUTES
COOKING TIME: 10 MINUTES

	Before	After
Calories	440	190
Fat (g)	18	2
Saturated Fat (g)	5	0
Sodium (mg)	660	600
Carbohydrate (g)	41	33
Fiber (g)	10	9
Protein (g)	29	11

Moms' Kitchen Notes: Serve with baked tortilla chips.

Slurry in a Hurry

If you want to thicken a soup or sauce without the addition of heavy cream or butter, try our Slurry in a Hurry. A slurry is a mixture of a cold liquid, such as broth or milk, and a starch, such as flour or cornstarch. When the mixture is whisked into a soup or heated in a skillet or saucepan, the starch granules absorb the liquid, thereby thickening the sauce or soup. The key to a successful slurry is . . .

- Making sure the starch is completely dissolved in the liquid before it is heated to avoid the starch forming unappetizing lumps.
- Stirring frequently as the mixture is heating to prevent the starch from sinking to the bottom of the pan where it will form a gluey mess.
- Cooking it for a few minutes to eliminate the starchy flavor.
- Using the right proportion of starch to liquid. For each 8-ounce cup of liquid, use 1 tablespoon of flour for a thin sauce, 2 tablespoons of flour for a medium sauce, and 3 tablespoons of flour for a thick sauce. Cornstarch has almost twice the thickening power as flour. Therefore, per cup of liquid, use about $\frac{1}{2}$ tablespoon for a thin sauce, 1 tablespoon for a medium sauce, and $1\frac{1}{2}$ tablespoons for a thick sauce.

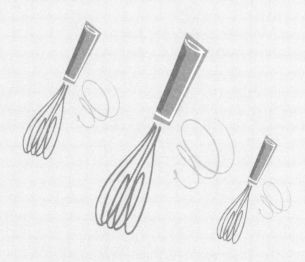

Corn & Carrot Chowder

MAKES 4 TO 5 SERVINGS

Okay. Let's get real. Who on earth has the time to make corn chowder by husking half a dozen ears of corn and then removing all the tiny kernels? Some corn chowder recipes ask you to do just that! To streamline this soup, we call for frozen corn kernels instead. And since we are self-described "overachievers," we also include carrots for extra color and nutrients.

Moms Make It Over By . . .

- Adding carrots for health-enhancing vitamins, minerals, phytonutrients, and fiber.
- Thickening the soup with lowfat milk and flour and eliminating the bacon to lower the saturated fat and calories.
- Using all-natural chicken broth to reduce the sodium.

> One 10-ounce bag or box frozen corn kernels (about 2 cups)
>
> 2 large carrots, shredded (about 2 cups), or 2 cups preshredded carrots
>
> 1 large baking potato, peeled and cut into ½-inch cubes (about 2 cups)
>
> 3 cups all-natural chicken broth or vegetable broth
>
> 1 bay leaf
>
> 1 teaspoon onion powder
>
> ¾ teaspoon dried thyme
>
> ½ teaspoon garlic powder
>
> 1 cup 1% lowfat milk
>
> 3 tablespoons all-purpose flour
>
> 1 tablespoon butter
>
> Salt and pepper
>
> ½ cup preshredded reduced-fat Cheddar cheese

1. Combine the corn, carrots, potato, broth, bay leaf, onion powder, thyme, and garlic powder in a large saucepan or Dutch oven and stir. Cover, and bring to a boil. Reduce the heat and simmer, covered, until the potatoes are tender, about 15 minutes.

2. Meanwhile, whisk together the milk and flour in a medium bowl until well blended.

3. When the potatoes are tender, stir in the milk mixture (rewhisk if necessary) and butter. Bring the soup back to a simmer, stirring constantly. Reduce the heat and continue to simmer and stir gently until the soup thickens slightly, about 2 minutes.

4. Remove the bay leaf and season with salt and pepper to taste. Serve in individual bowls and top with the cheese.

PREPARATION TIME: 15 MINUTES
COOKING TIME: 20 MINUTES

	Before	After
Calories	360	240
Fat (g)	14	5
Saturated Fat (g)	8	2.5
Sodium (mg)	1,010	540
Carbohydrate (g)	46	42
Fiber (g)	5	5
Protein (g)	15	11

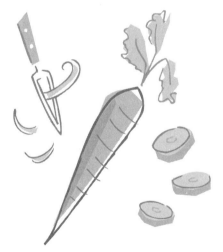

Salmon Seashell Chowder

MAKES 4 SERVINGS

Clams are a good source of healthy omega-3 fats, but salmon is even better! That fact motivated us to retool the classic cream-laden recipe for New England clam chowder using salmon instead. Making this soup from scratch is easy thanks to boneless pink salmon, now available in convenient no-fuss pouches.

Moms Make It Over By ...

- Adding peas for vitamins, minerals, phytonutrients, and fiber.
- Switching to salmon for even more healthy omega-3 fats.
- Thickening the soup with lowfat milk and flour to lower the saturated fat and calories.
- Using all-natural chicken broth to reduce the sodium.

   4 ounces dried medium pasta shells (about 1½ cups)

   2 cups 1% lowfat milk

   1 cup all-natural chicken broth

   3 tablespoons all-purpose flour

   1 teaspoon onion powder

   ¾ teaspoon dried dill

   1½ cups frozen peas, thawed

   One 7-ounce pouch skinless, boneless pink salmon, flaked

   Salt and pepper

1. Cook the pasta according to package directions. Drain and set aside.

2. In a saucepan, combine the milk, broth, flour, onion powder, and dill and whisk until well blended. Add the peas and salmon, and place the saucepan over high heat. Bring the mixture to a simmer, stirring constantly. Reduce the heat and continue to simmer and stir gently until the soup thickens slightly, about 2 minutes.

3. Stir in the pasta and season with salt and pepper to taste. Heat through and serve.

PREPARATION TIME: 5 MINUTES
COOKING TIME: 20 MINUTES

Moms' Kitchen Notes: If you can't find salmon in a pouch, then use a 6-ounce can of skinless, boneless pink salmon.

	Before	After
Calories	480	280
Fat (g)	29	4
Saturated Fat (g)	16	2
Sodium (mg)	1,100	520
Carbohydrate (g)	25	40
Fiber (g)	2	3
Protein (g)	28	20

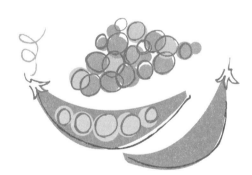

Orange Soup

The last time Liz made butternut squash soup, she wished she had a machete because slicing the rock-hard squash nearly destroyed her chef's knife. Winter squash are bursting with health-enhancing beta-carotene as well as great flavor . . . but they're a pain to prepare. Our version of butternut squash soup relies on frozen squash and carrots so the prep is a breeze. Sure, you still have to cook it, but now you have extra time with the kids.

Moms Make It Over By . . .

- Adding carrots for vitamins, minerals, phytonutrients, and fiber.
- Using all-natural chicken broth to lower the sodium.

> One 20-ounce bag frozen butternut squash
>
> 2¼ cups all-natural chicken broth or vegetable broth
>
> 2 cups frozen carrots
>
> ½ cup orange juice
>
> 1 tablespoon pure maple syrup
>
> ½ teaspoon ground cinnamon
>
> ½ teaspoon garlic powder
>
> ¼ teaspoon ground ginger
>
> Pinch ground cloves
>
> ½ cup reduced-fat sour cream
>
> ½ cup seasoned croutons

1. Combine the butternut squash, broth, carrots, orange juice, maple syrup, cinnamon, garlic powder, ginger, and cloves in a large saucepan or Dutch oven and stir. Cover and bring to a boil. Reduce the heat and simmer, covered, until the carrots are tender, 15 to 20 minutes.

2. Transfer the soup to a food processor or blender and process until smooth. Work in batches if necessary. Return the soup to the pan and whisk in the sour cream. Reheat if necessary.

3. Serve in individual bowls and top with the croutons.

PREPARATION TIME: 5 MINUTES
COOKING TIME: 25 MINUTES

Moms′ Kitchen Notes: Other topping ideas include toasted and chopped walnuts or pecans, and shredded reduced-fat Cheddar cheese.

	Before	After
Calories	230	200
Fat (g)	11	5
Saturated Fat (g)	5	2.5
Sodium (mg)	1,150	430
Carbohydrate (g)	31	37
Fiber (g)	4	4
Protein (g)	4	5

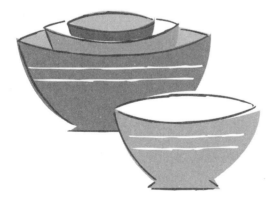

Kale, Sweet Potato, & Kielbasa Soup

MAKES 6 TO 8 SERVINGS

From now on when you hear the word "kale" think "K" for vitamin K . . . a little-known nutrient important for bone health. The idea for this recipe came from a mom who knew that the kale and sweet potatoes in her soup were nutritional bonanzas but kind of questioned the high-fat kielbasa.

Moms Make It Over By . . .

- Switching to low-fat kielbasa to lower the saturated fat and calories.
- Using all-natural chicken broth to reduce the sodium.

1 tablespoon olive oil

1 medium onion, finely chopped (about 1 cup), or 1 cup frozen chopped onion

2 large sweet potatoes, peeled and cut into ½-inch cubes (about 6 cups)

Two 10-ounce boxes or one 16-ounce bag frozen chopped kale or spinach

One 14- or 16-ounce package low-fat kielbasa, sliced into ¼-inch rounds

One 32-ounce carton all-natural chicken broth (4 cups)

1 tablespoon brown sugar

½ teaspoon ground cinnamon

1. Heat the oil in a large saucepan or Dutch oven over medium-high heat. Add the onion and cook until translucent, about 5 minutes.

2. Add the sweet potatoes, kale, kielbasa, broth, 1 cup water, sugar, and cinnamon and stir to combine. Cover and bring to a boil. Reduce the heat and simmer, covered, until the sweet potatoes are tender, 20 to 25 minutes.

	Before	After
Calories	360	190
Fat (g)	26	7
Saturated Fat (g)	8	1.5
Sodium (mg)	1,590	850
Carbohydrate (g)	22	22
Fiber (g)	3	4
Protein (g)	13	12

PREPARATION TIME: **15 MINUTES**
COOKING TIME: **30 MINUTES**

Moms' Kitchen Notes: Serve with Honey Wheat Popovers (page 308).

Shrimpy Green Coconut Soup

MAKES 4 TO 5 SERVINGS

Collard greens are one of those supercharged vegetables—rich in vitamin K and carotenoids—so we just had to find a place for them in our book. Though we're not quite sure how we came up with the idea of adding collard greens to Thai coconut soup, we can honestly say that it's one of our favorites.

Moms Make It Over By ...

- Adding collard greens for vitamins, minerals, phytonutrients, and fiber.
- Switching to lite coconut milk to lower the saturated fat and calories.
- Eliminating the fish sauce and using all-natural chicken broth to reduce the sodium.

One 32-ounce carton all-natural chicken broth (4 cups)

One 14-ounce can lite coconut milk

One 10-ounce box frozen collard greens or spinach (about 2 cups)

$^2/_3$ cup jasmine rice

2 tablespoons bottled or fresh lime juice

2 teaspoons bottled minced ginger or $^1/_2$ teaspoon ground ginger

1 teaspoon dried curry powder

One 4-ounce can tiny cocktail shrimp, drained and rinsed

1. Combine the broth, coconut milk, collard greens, rice, lime juice, ginger, and curry powder in a large saucepan or Dutch oven and stir. Cover and bring to a boil. Reduce the heat and cook at a low boil until the rice is cooked, about 20 minutes.

2. Stir in the shrimp, heat through, and serve.

PREPARATION TIME: 5 MINUTES

COOKING TIME: 25 MINUTES

	Before	After
Calories	460	230
Fat (g)	38	7
Saturated Fat (g)	30	4.5
Sodium (mg)	2,500	720
Carbohydrate (g)	6	33
Fiber (g)	2	3
Protein (g)	27	11

Cheesy Broccoli Soup

MAKES 4 TO 5 SERVINGS

A lot of health-conscious moms shy away from cream of vegetable soups because they're loaded with fat. Hey, we can't blame them. And when you consider that just ½ cup of heavy cream has over 400 calories and 44 grams of fat, it's easy to see why. Our easy makeover nixes the heavy cream without losing the creaminess of the soup.

Moms Make It Over By . . .

🍓 Using lowfat milk and reduced-fat cheese to lower the saturated fat.

2½ cups all-natural chicken broth or vegetable broth

One 16-ounce package broccoli cuts or spears

2½ cups 1% lowfat milk

3 tablespoons all-purpose flour

1 teaspoon onion powder

1 teaspoon garlic powder

1 teaspoon Dijon mustard

1 cup preshredded reduced-fat Cheddar cheese

Salt and pepper

¼ cup Parmesan cheese, optional

1. Place the broth and broccoli in a large saucepan or Dutch oven over high heat. Cover, bring to a boil, and cook until the broccoli is tender, about 5 minutes.

2. Transfer the mixture to a food processor or blender and process until smooth. Return to the pan and place over medium-high heat.

3. Meanwhile, whisk together the milk, flour, onion powder, garlic powder, and mustard in a large bowl until well blended. Stir the mixture into the pureed broccoli and bring to a simmer, stirring constantly. Reduce the heat and continue to simmer and stir gently until the soup thickens, about 2 minutes.

4. Add the Cheddar cheese and stir until melted. Season with salt and pepper to taste. Serve in individual bowls and top with Parmesan cheese as desired.

Moms' Kitchen Notes: Serve with Carrot-Top Tuna (page 125).

	Before	After
Calories	160	150
Fat (g)	13	3.5
Saturated Fat (g)	7	2
Sodium (mg)	690	580
Carbohydrate (g)	8	17
Fiber (g)	3	3
Protein (g)	4	15

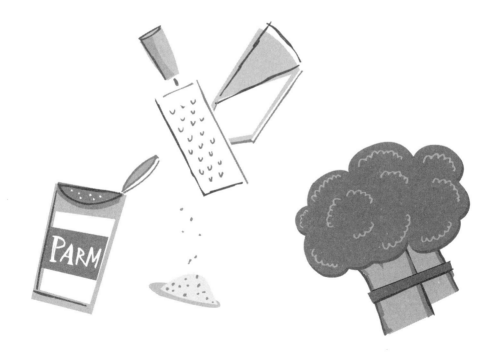

Chicken Stew with Baby Carrots

MAKES 4 TO 6 SERVINGS

Our deliciously simple chicken stew is a takeoff on Chicken Fricassee . . . a classic French dish where chicken—skin and all—is sautéed in butter before it's stewed with vegetables. At over 600 calories in a serving, we figured a recipe rescue was in order. You'll appreciate the shortcuts we use in preparing this weeknight dish, but don't expect it on the table in minutes. Stews require some serious stove time so the flavors have a chance to meld.

Moms Make It Over By . . .

- Adding carrots and mushrooms for vitamins, minerals, phytonutrients, and fiber.
- Using skinless, boneless chicken breast and cooking in a moderate amount of healthy olive oil to lower the saturated fat and calories.
- Cutting the salt to reduce the sodium.

> 1½ pounds skinless, boneless chicken breast halves, each cut into 3 pieces
>
> ¼ cup all-purpose flour
>
> 1 tablespoon olive oil
>
> One 10-ounce package presliced mushrooms
>
> 1 teaspoon bottled crushed garlic, or 1 to 2 garlic cloves, minced
>
> 1½ cups all-natural chicken broth
>
> One 16-ounce bag ready-to-eat baby carrots, or one 16-ounce bag frozen baby carrots, thawed
>
> One 8-ounce can tomato sauce
>
> ½ cup kalamata olives, coarsely chopped, or one 2¼-ounce can sliced olives, drained, optional
>
> 1 teaspoon Italian seasoning
>
> Salt and pepper

1. Place the chicken and flour in a bowl and toss to coat the chicken evenly. Shake off excess flour.

2. Heat the oil in a large saucepan or Dutch oven over medium-high heat. Add the chicken and cook, turning a few times, until lightly browned, about 3 minutes.

3. Add the mushrooms, garlic, and a few tablespoons of the broth. Cook, stirring occasionally, until the mushrooms are tender, about 5 minutes. If the chicken sticks to the pan, add additional broth, loosening up any brown bits from the bottom.

4. Stir in the carrots, the remaining broth, tomato sauce, olives as desired, and Italian seasoning. Cover and bring to a boil. Reduce the heat and simmer, covered, 20 minutes. Remove the cover and simmer until the carrots are tender and the stew thickens, an additional 10 to 15 minutes.

5. Season with salt and pepper to taste and serve.

PREPARATION TIME: 15 MINUTES
COOKING TIME: 40 TO 45 MINUTES

Moms' Kitchen Notes: Serve with polenta or pasta.

	Before	After
Calories	630	260
Fat (g)	37	6
Saturated Fat (g)	16	1.5
Sodium (mg)	1,430	580
Carbohydrate (g)	19	20
Fiber (g)	3	3
Protein (g)	53	31

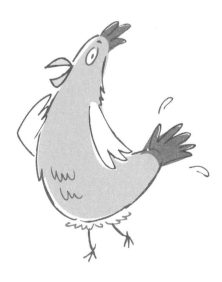

Halftime Taco Chili

MAKES 6 SERVINGS

Janice went to her sister Lori's house for Super Bowl Sunday one year and barely watched the game because she was too busy sampling the halftime food spread. One of her favorite dishes on the table was her sister's signature taco chili, but when Janice learned what was in it—taco seasoning mix, Ranch dressing mix, and beef bouillon—the sodium alone blew her away. Our new-and-improved version scores a touchdown for good nutrition.

Moms Make It Over By . . .

- Adding carrots for vitamins, minerals, phytonutrients, and fiber.
- Switching to lean ground beef to lower the saturated fat and calories.
- Replacing the packets of Ranch dressing and taco seasoning with a flavorful blend of spices and seasonings to reduce the sodium.

1 tablespoon canola oil

2 large carrots, shredded (about 2 cups)

1 medium onion, coarsely chopped (about 1 cup), or 1 cup frozen chopped onion

1 pound lean ground beef (90% or higher)

One 28-ounce can crushed tomatoes

One 15½-ounce can black-eyed peas or pinto beans, drained and rinsed

One 15-ounce can yellow or white hominy, drained and rinsed

One 4-ounce can diced green chili peppers, optional

2 to 3 teaspoons chili powder

2 to 3 teaspoons ground cumin

1 teaspoon garlic powder

½ cup reduced-fat sour cream

⅓ cup preshredded reduced-fat Cheddar cheese

1. Heat the oil in a large saucepan or Dutch oven over medium-high heat.

2. Add the carrots, onion, and beef and cook, breaking up the large pieces, until the meat is no longer pink, 5 to 7 minutes. Drain excess fat.

3. Stir in the tomatoes, black-eyed peas, hominy, 1 cup water, chili peppers as desired, chili powder, cumin, and garlic powder and bring to a boil. Reduce the heat and simmer, covered, until the carrots are tender, 20 to 25 minutes.

4. Remove from the heat and stir in the sour cream. Serve in individual bowls and top with shredded cheese.

PREPARATION TIME: **15 MINUTES**
COOKING TIME: **30 MINUTES**

	Before	After
Calories	410	340
Fat (g)	18	10
Saturated Fat (g)	6	3.5
Sodium (mg)	1,520	570
Carbohydrate (g)	38	37
Fiber (g)	7	8
Protein (g)	23	27

Moms′ Kitchen Notes: If you can't find hominy near the canned vegetables or canned beans in your grocery store, substitute 2 cups frozen corn kernels.

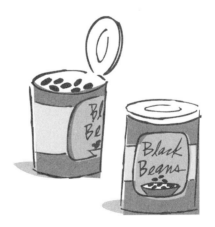

White Bean Cassoulet Soup

MAKES 6 SERVINGS

If you lived in France, cassoulet would probably be on your list of family favorites. This classic mouthwatering meal from southwest France is made with white beans and various meats, including sausage, pork, and duck cooked in its own fat. It can take days to prepare and have nearly a day's worth of saturated fat in a serving. We're not kidding. To say au revoir to the cooking time and most of the unhealthy fat, we created our own fast and delicious version sans the fatty meats.

Moms Make It Over By . . .

- Adding lima beans and carrots for vitamins, minerals, phytonutrients, and fiber.
- Using light breakfast sausage to lower the saturated fat and calories.
- Using all-natural chicken broth to reduce the sodium.

One 32-ounce carton all-natural chicken broth (4 cups)

One 15½-ounce can cannellini beans, drained and rinsed

One 14-ounce can diced tomatoes

1 cup frozen baby lima beans or edamame beans, thawed

One 8-ounce package frozen, precooked light breakfast sausage, thawed and thinly sliced

2 large carrots, shredded (about 2 cups), or 2 cups preshredded carrots

¾ teaspoon onion powder

¾ teaspoon garlic powder

¼ teaspoon dried thyme and/or ¼ teaspoon dried rosemary

¼ cup grated Parmesan cheese

1. Combine the broth, cannellini beans, tomatoes, lima beans, sausage, carrots, onion powder, garlic powder, and thyme in a large saucepan or Dutch oven and stir. Cover and bring to a boil. Reduce the heat and cook at a low boil, covered, until the carrots are tender, about 15 minutes.

2. Serve in individual bowls and top with Parmesan cheese.

PREPARATION TIME: 15 MINUTES

COOKING TIME: 20 MINUTES

	Before	After
Calories	890	210
Fat (g)	42	8
Saturated Fat (g)	14	3
Sodium (mg)	1,880	830
Carbohydrate (g)	64	22
Fiber (g)	17	6
Protein (g)	57	13

CHAPTER 6

Smart Sandwiches & Wraps

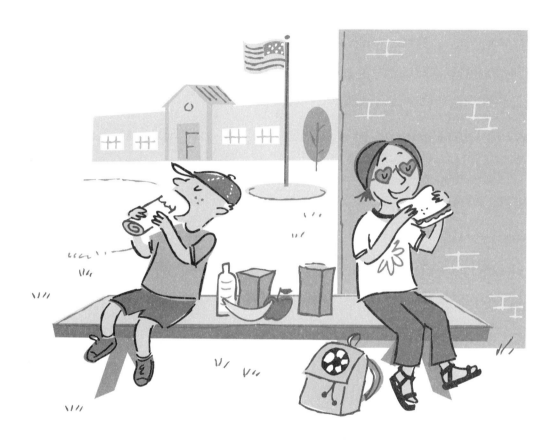

Carrot-Top Tuna • Ham & Cheese Pinwheels • Colorful Sweet Potato Burritos • Popeye's Veggie Pitas • Gotta-Have Grilled Cheese • Grape-Nuts Chicken Salad • Broc 'n Roll Wraps • Reuben Reinvented • Super Sloppy Joes • Healthy Hero • Turkey All Wrapped Up • The Full Monte Cristo

No matter how you slice them, Americans love sandwiches. In fact, as a nation, we eat more than 45 billion sandwiches each year. In 1762, when John Montague, the fourth Earl of Sandwich, ordered two pieces of bread with meat in between, the sandwich was born. Back then, who would have guessed that the sandwich would ultimately become a familiar staple in our diets?

When we were growing up, a quick sandwich with potato chips and a pickle on the side was the standard lunchtime fare. The choices were pretty limited back then to grilled cheese—cooked in a skillet full of melted butter (yum!)—tuna salad on white, and ham or bologna and cheese with an ample dollop of mayo. Happily, today a new generation of sandwiches has given rise to things like grilled Portobello mushrooms with goat cheese and roasted red bell peppers on focaccia bread. Okay, maybe that's a bit too sophisticated for some young palates, but between the different types of breads, condiments, and fillings now available, the sandwich has graduated to a more interesting and, if you make the right choices, healthy meal option.

Building a better sandwich for today's health-conscious families is easy. All it takes is a few additions, subtractions, and substitutions from the tried-and-true favorites. You'll notice that we don't use white sandwich bread in our recipes. Instead, we have opted for the 100% whole wheat and whole grain bread varieties that provide more nutrients and fiber. Given the fact that on average, Americans only eat one whole grain food a day despite the recommendation to eat at least three, we thought it was a pretty smart idea. Mayonnaise is still a staple in some of our recipes, but we suggest using a light canola mayonnaise to slim things down a bit while still getting important omega-3 fats into the meal (canola oil contains more omega-3s than most other oils). Our Grape-Nuts Chicken Salad (page 133) is the perfect example of how a sandwich, once swimming in creamy mayonnaise, is now bursting with flavor and health. The chicken gets tossed with grapes and toasted pecans and mixed with a small amount of light canola mayo before it's stuffed into a high-energy, high-fiber whole wheat pita half.

As you read this chapter you'll discover tricks for adding more delicious vegetables to sandwiches, adding pizzazz to the same old turkey and cheese, and reinventing classic sandwiches like the Reuben to have half the fat and sodium as the original. Each recipe offers new ways to transform the simple sandwich into a fast and nourishing weekday or weeknight meal. After all, moms deserve a break from time to time, so turn to sandwiches to make your life a little bit easier.

Carrot-Top Tuna

MAKES 6 SERVINGS

If you're trying to get your kids hooked on more heart-healthy seafood, turn to tuna. But the tuna sandwich of years gone by (and even today) was typically made with a boatload of full-fat mayonnaise, white bread, and little else. Our clever makeover weaves in both a fruit and a vegetable, pleasing Mom and the kids.

Moms Make It Over By . . .

- Adding carrot and apple for vitamins, minerals, phytonutrients, and fiber.
- Using water-packed tuna and light canola mayonnaise to lower the calories.
- Using whole wheat bread for added nutrients and fiber.

Two 6-ounce cans solid white tuna in water, drained and flaked

1 large carrot, shredded (about 1 cup), or 1 cup preshredded carrots

1 medium Granny Smith apple, peeled, cored, and coarsely chopped (about 1 cup)

½ cup light canola mayonnaise

1 tablespoon honey mustard

12 slices whole wheat bread, toasted if desired

1. Combine the tuna, carrot, apple, mayonnaise, and honey mustard in a medium bowl and mix well.

2. Spread the tuna mixture evenly over each of 6 bread slices. Top with the remaining bread slices. Cut in half and serve.

PREPARATION TIME: 15 MINUTES

Moms' Kitchen Notes: For even more fiber and flavor, add ½ cup golden raisins and/or ½ cup chopped walnuts.

	Before	After
Calories	450	280
Fat (g)	27	9
Saturated Fat (g)	4	1
Sodium (mg)	770	600
Carbohydrate (g)	25	33
Fiber (g)	1	5
Protein (g)	26	19

Ham & Cheese Pinwheels

MAKES 4 SERVINGS

The ham sandwich has been the number one American favorite for more than a decade. Made by simply placing a few slices of ham and cheese between two slices of white bread and slathering them with mayonnaise—what could be easier? Besides our obvious mission to cut the saturated fat and sodium, we modernized the old classic by adding some surprising ingredients, including carrots for cancer-fighting carotenoids.

Moms Make It Over By . . .

- Adding carrots for vitamins, minerals, phytonutrients, and fiber.
- Switching to lean deli ham and reduced-fat cheese to lower the saturated fat, calories, and sodium.
- Using whole wheat flour tortillas for added nutrients and fiber.

½ cup light cream cheese, softened

Four 8-inch whole wheat flour tortillas

1 large carrot, shredded (about 1 cup), or 1 cup preshredded carrots

½ cup preshredded reduced-fat Cheddar cheese

6 ounces thinly sliced lean deli ham

DIPPING SAUCES

¼ cup honey mustard

¼ cup barbecue sauce

¼ cup hummus

1. Spread the cream cheese evenly over each of the tortillas.

2. Layer each tortilla with carrots, Cheddar cheese, and ham.

3. Roll up tightly and slice into ¾-inch rounds. Serve with your choice of dipping sauces.

PREPARATION TIME: 15 MINUTES

Moms' Kitchen Notes: For a school lunch option, slice the wrap in half and include your child's favorite dipping sauce in a small plastic container on the side.

	Before	After
Calories	450	290
Fat (g)	27	9
Saturated Fat (g)	10	5
Sodium (mg)	1,560	880
Carbohydrate (g)	30	42
Fiber (g)	1	4
Protein (g)	20	19

PB&J: More Than a Lunch box Favorite

There's no denying the fact that the peanut butter & jelly sandwich is the unparalleled king of all kid sandwiches. But adults love it, too. In fact, Elvis Presley was a big fan . . . his favorite was peanut butter and banana on white bread! If your children are in a PB&J rut, you'll applaud our updated Elvis-inspired recipes, bursting with extra fiber, flavor, and nutrients.

The Jail House Rock: Peanut butter & sliced Granny Smith apples on whole wheat bread
The Hound Dog: Peanut butter, raisins, & banana on whole wheat pita
The All Shook Up: Almond butter & all-fruit strawberry jam on whole wheat bread
The Don't Be Cruel: Soy nut butter & all-fruit apricot jam on a whole wheat tortilla

Colorful Sweet Potato Burritos

MAKES 6 TO 8 SERVINGS

Fast food burritos filled with meat, refried beans, cheese, and sour cream have become almost as popular as burgers and fries . . . and almost as high in saturated fat and calories. We say, "Why bother, when you can make 'em yourself." If you're looking for a no-stress solution to feeding your family more veggies, our easy burritos—made with one of nature's most kid-pleasing, antioxidant-rich vegetables—are the answer.

Moms Make It Over By . . .

- Adding sweet potatoes, corn, and salsa for vitamins, minerals, phytonutrients, and fiber.
- Switching to fat-free refried beans, reduced-fat sour cream, and reduced-fat cheese to lower the saturated fat and calories.

1 large sweet potato, peeled and cut into ½-inch cubes (about 3 cups)

One 16-ounce can fat-free refried beans

Eight 8-inch flour tortillas

1½ cups preshredded reduced-fat Cheddar cheese

1 cup frozen corn kernels, thawed

½ to 1 cup salsa

½ cup reduced-fat sour cream

1 ripe avocado, peeled, pitted, and sliced, optional

1. Steam the sweet potato until tender, about 8 minutes. Set aside.

2. Lightly oil or coat a large baking sheet with nonstick cooking spray and set aside.

3. Preheat the oven to 375°F.

4. Spread the refried beans evenly over each of 8 tortillas and sprinkle with the cheese. Arrange the sweet potato, corn, and salsa evenly down the center of each.

5. Roll up burrito-style and place seam side down on the baking sheet. Bake until the cheese melts and the burritos are heated through, about 15 minutes. Serve with sour cream and avocado as desired.

PREPARATION TIME: 20 MINUTES
COOKING TIME: 15 MINUTES

Moms' Kitchen Notes: To streamline the prep time, steam the sweet potatoes the night before.

	Before	After
Calories	500	340
Fat (g)	20	7
Saturated Fat (g)	7	2.5
Sodium (mg)	1,660	740
Carbohydrate (g)	51	54
Fiber (g)	3	8
Protein (g)	27	14

Popeye's Veggie Pitas

MAKES 4 SERVINGS

Of all the vegetables Americans eat, green leafy vegetables account for just 3 percent . . . a mere pittance compared to iceberg lettuce at 16 percent. That's unfortunate because eating green every day can lower our risk of certain cancers, help maintain strong bones and teeth, and keep eyes healthy as we age. All of those benefits, plus the fact that green leafy vegetables taste great, were reason enough to stuff spinach into these delicious veggie pitas.

Moms Make It Over By . . .

- Adding spinach and bell pepper for vitamins, minerals, phytonutrients, and fiber.
- Switching to a smaller portion of part-skim cheese to lower the saturated fat and calories.
- Using whole wheat pita pockets and including hummus for added nutrients and fiber.

    2 cups packed baby spinach

    2 tablespoons lite or regular Caesar salad dressing

    2 large whole wheat pitas, halved

    ½ cup hummus

    1 small red bell pepper, thinly sliced

    4 ounces thinly sliced part-skim mozzarella cheese

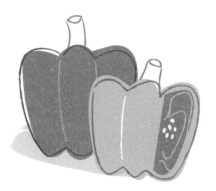

1. Combine the spinach and salad dressing in a medium bowl and mix well.

2. Line each pita pocket evenly with the hummus, bell pepper, spinach, and cheese and serve.

PREPARATION TIME: 10 MINUTES

Moms' Kitchen Notes: If your children don't like bell peppers, switch to shredded carrots or sliced tomatoes instead.

	Before	After
Calories	570	230
Fat (g)	32	9
Saturated Fat (g)	18	3.5
Sodium (mg)	800	560
Carbohydrate (g)	49	26
Fiber (g)	4	5
Protein (g)	23	14

Gotta-Have Grilled Cheese

MAKES 4 SERVINGS

When we need a last-minute meal that the kids will eat without a fuss, we invariably turn to grilled cheese. The classic recipe (if you'd even call it a recipe) calls for white bread, a few slices of processed American cheese, and a generous amount of butter. But with nearly a day's worth of saturated fat in one little sandwich, a recipe rescue was inevitable.

Moms Make It Over By . . .

- Adding tomatoes for vitamins, minerals, phytonutrients, and fiber.
- Switching to part-skim cheese and cooking in a moderate amount of healthy canola oil to lower the saturated fat and calories.
- Using whole wheat bread for added nutrients and fiber.

> 8 slices 100% whole wheat bread
>
> 6 ounces thinly sliced part-skim mozzarella cheese
>
> 8 paper-thin tomato slices
>
> 1 tablespoon canola oil

1. Top each of 4 bread slices evenly with the cheese and tomatoes and place the remaining bread slices firmly on top.

2. Heat half the oil in a large nonstick skillet over medium-high heat.

3. Add the sandwiches and cook until the bottoms are golden brown, 2 to 3 minutes. Add the remaining oil, flip the sandwiches, and cook until the cheese melts, an additional 2 to 3 minutes. Slice and serve warm.

PREPARATION TIME: 10 MINUTES

COOKING TIME: 5 MINUTES

	Before	After
Calories	480	290
Fat (g)	35	13
Saturated Fat (g)	21	6
Sodium (mg)	1,230	520
Carbohydrate (g)	26	28
Fiber (g)	1	4
Protein (g)	17	17

Grape-Nuts Chicken Salad

MAKES 4 SERVINGS

When Liz was a teen, she worked in a sandwich shop where chicken salad was the specialty. If the customers ever knew how much mayonnaise the cook used in each sandwich, they would have been shocked. . . . Liz certainly was. To assuage her guilt for serving all those fat-laden sandwiches, Liz created this light and easy Grape-Nuts Chicken Salad sandwich, where grapes and pecans add family-friendly appeal . . . with half the calories.

Moms Make It Over By . . .

- Adding grapes for vitamins, minerals, phytonutrients, and fiber.
- Including pecans for added nutrients and heart-healthy monounsaturated fats.
- Using whole wheat pita for added nutrients and fiber.

12 ounces cooked chicken breast, coarsely chopped

⅔ cup seedless green grapes, quartered

⅓ cup pecans, toasted and coarsely chopped

½ cup light canola mayonnaise

½ teaspoon dried tarragon

¼ teaspoon salt

Pepper

2 large whole wheat pitas, halved

1. Combine the chicken, grapes, pecans, mayonnaise, tarragon, salt, and pepper to taste in a large bowl and mix well.

2. Add the chicken mixture to each of the pita halves and serve.

PREPARATION TIME: 15 MINUTES

	Before	After
Calories	470	380
Fat (g)	32	17
Saturated Fat (g)	5	1.5
Sodium (mg)	740	500
Carbohydrate (g)	26	26
Fiber (g)	2	4
Protein (g)	18	31

Moms' Kitchen Notes: For the cooked chicken in this dish, use leftovers or bake skinless, boneless chicken breast halves at 350°F for about 20 minutes.

Broc 'n Roll Wraps

MAKES 4 SERVINGS

A recent stroll down the supermarket frozen food aisle revealed that although some of today's frozen pocket sandwiches seem nutritious, names can be misleading. Take one of the healthiest-sounding pockets: Chicken, Cheddar & Broccoli. When we read the label, we discovered it contained zero percent of vitamins A and C . . . a clue that the pockets had a negligible amount of broccoli. Our homemade version is the real deal with 35 percent of vitamin A and 80 percent of vitamin C.

Moms Make It Over By . . .

- Adding broccoli for vitamins, minerals, phytonutrients, and fiber.
- Using reduced-fat cheese to lower the saturated fat and calories.
- Using whole wheat flour tortillas for added nutrients and fiber.

> **3 cups fresh or frozen broccoli florets**
> **Four 8-inch whole wheat flour tortillas**
> **1⅓ cups preshredded reduced-fat Cheddar cheese**

1. Steam the broccoli until very tender, 5 to 7 minutes. Set aside.

2. One at a time, place each tortilla on a plate, top with ⅓ cup cheese, and heat in the microwave oven until the cheese melts, about 40 seconds.

3. Arrange the broccoli evenly down the center of each tortilla. Gently break up the broccoli using the back of a fork.

4. Roll up, slice in half, and serve.

PREPARATION TIME: 10 MINUTES

	Before	After
Calories	320	200
Fat (g)	14	3.5
Saturated Fat (g)	6	2
Sodium (mg)	560	520
Carbohydrate (g)	38	36
Fiber (g)	3	5
Protein (g)	10	15

Whole Wheat Bread: Be 100% Sure

Whole wheat bread is a good source of fiber, vitamin E, zinc, and other important phytonutrients. That's because it's made with the bran and germ layers of the wheat kernel where most of the nutrients reside. White bread, or for that matter, "wheat" bread, is made with refined flour in which the bran and germ have been removed. Although the government requires that refined flour be enriched with some of the nutrients that were stripped away, things like fiber are not added back. In fact, 75 percent of the vitamins, minerals, and phytonutrients found in whole grains are lost when they're refined.

To choose the best bread:

- Make sure it says "100% whole wheat" on the label.
- Look for the words "whole wheat flour" as the first ingredient listed.
- Don't be misled by words such as "wheat," "stoneground," "cracked wheat" or "unbleached wheat," because they are not the same as 100% whole wheat or whole grain.
- Expect to find 2 or more grams of fiber in every slice of 100% whole wheat bread.

Even if you buy 7-grain or multigrain bread, there's no guarantee you're getting a high-fiber option because the first ingredient listed could still be "enriched wheat," aka refined flour.

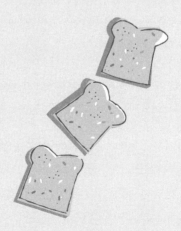

Reuben Reinvented

MAKES 4 SERVINGS

The name Arthur Reuben may not ring a bell, but he's the deli owner credited with inventing the Reuben sandwich. Made with generous amounts of corned beef, Swiss cheese, sauerkraut, and Russian dressing jammed between two slices of rye bread and grilled in butter, the original sandwich had more fat than a Big Mac. Hey Arthur, what were you thinking?

Moms Make It Over By . . .

- Switching to light canola mayonnaise, reduced-fat cheese, and lean deli corned beef, and cooking in a moderate amount of healthy canola oil to lower the saturated fat and calories.
- Using coleslaw instead of sauerkraut for greater kid appeal and half the sodium.

> 1½ cups preshredded coleslaw mix
> 3 tablespoons light canola mayonnaise
> 1 tablespoon Dijon mustard
> 8 slices rye bread
> 4 ounces thinly sliced, reduced-fat Swiss cheese
> 4 ounces thinly sliced lean deli corned beef
> 1 tablespoon canola oil

1. Combine the coleslaw, mayonnaise, and mustard in a medium bowl and mix well.

2. Top each of 4 bread slices evenly with the cheese, coleslaw mixture, and corned beef. Place the remaining bread slices firmly on top.

3. Heat half the oil in a large nonstick skillet over medium-high heat. Add the sandwiches and cook until the bottoms are golden brown, 2 to 3 minutes.

4. Add the remaining oil, flip the sandwiches, and cook until the cheese melts, an additional 2 to 3 minutes. Slice and serve warm.

	Before	After
Calories	590	320
Fat (g)	38	15
Saturated Fat (g)	15	5
Sodium (mg)	1,860	780
Carbohydrate (g)	36	29
Fiber (g)	6	4
Protein (g)	25	18

Moms' Kitchen Notes: Serve with baby carrots.

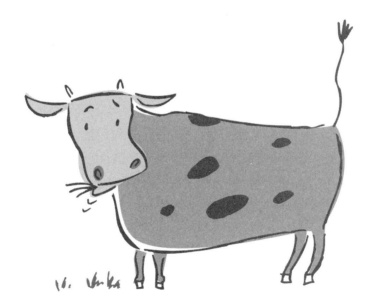

Super Sloppy Joes

MAKES 6 SERVINGS

Serving Sloppy Joes for dinner is a great excuse to make a mess at the table! It's also a great excuse to add a vegetable to your family's diet. Although Sloppy Joes are traditionally made with ground beef, a tomato-based sauce, and a big hamburger bun, we took creative license by enhancing our sloppy sauce with a finely diced bell pepper. The result: over half a day's supply of vitamins A and C as well as cancer-fighting carotenoids.

Moms Make It Over By . . .

- Adding bell pepper for vitamins, minerals, phytonutrients, and fiber.
- Switching to lean ground beef to lower the saturated fat.
- Using whole wheat hamburger buns for added nutrients and fiber.

> 1 tablespoon olive oil
>
> 1 large red or yellow bell pepper, finely diced (about 1½ cups)
>
> 1 small onion, finely chopped (about ½ cup)
>
> 1¼ pounds lean ground beef or turkey (90% lean or higher)
>
> ½ teaspoon garlic powder
>
> One 26-ounce jar pasta sauce
>
> 6 whole wheat hamburger buns, halved and toasted
>
> 6 tablespoons grated Parmesan cheese

1. Heat the oil in a large nonstick skillet over medium-high heat.

2. Add the bell pepper and onion and cook until tender, 5 to 7 minutes.

3. Add the beef and garlic powder and cook, breaking up the large pieces, until the meat is no longer pink, about 5 minutes. Drain excess fat.

4. Add the pasta sauce, reduce the heat, and simmer until heated through, 3 to 5 minutes.

5. Serve open-face-style over hamburger buns and top with Parmesan cheese.

PREPARATION TIME: 10 MINUTES
COOKING TIME: 15 MINUTES

Moms' Kitchen Notes: If you can't find whole wheat hamburger buns, ask your supermarket to stock them. The more you ask, the more likely they are to carry them.

	Before	After
Calories	380	330
Fat (g)	17	11
Saturated Fat (g)	6	3.5
Sodium (mg)	790	740
Carbohydrate (g)	35	34
Fiber (g)	2	6
Protein (g)	21	27

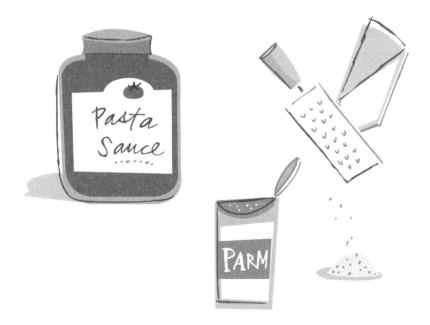

Healthy Hero

No matter what you call it—grinder, hoagie, submarine, or hero—this huge sandwich, loaded with sliced deli meats, cheese, tomatoes, pickles, and dressing is often so thick it's hard to take that very first bite. Our Healthy Hero is easier to eat and a whole lot lighter than the original version.

Moms Make It Over By . . .

- Adding spinach and tomato for vitamins, minerals, phytonutrients, and fiber.
- Switching to roasted turkey and reduced-fat cheese to lower the saturated fat, calories, and sodium.
- Using whole wheat submarine rolls for added nutrients and fiber.

2 cups packed baby spinach or romaine lettuce

2 tablespoons lite or regular Italian salad dressing

4 teaspoons honey mustard

4 whole wheat submarine rolls, halved

4 ounces thinly sliced roast beef

4 ounces thinly sliced reduced-fat Provolone cheese

4 ounces thinly sliced roasted turkey

4 sandwich-cut dill pickles

1 medium tomato, thinly sliced

1. Combine the spinach and salad dressing in a medium bowl and mix well.

2. Spread a teaspoon of the mustard on one side of each roll. Layer evenly with the spinach, roast beef, cheese, turkey, pickle, and tomato. Place the remaining roll halves firmly on top. Slice in half and serve.

PREPARATION TIME: 10 MINUTES

	Before	After
Calories	620	360
Fat (g)	35	12
Saturated Fat (g)	15	5
Sodium (mg)	1,860	880
Carbohydrate (g)	47	41
Fiber (g)	4	6
Protein (g)	27	29

Turkey All Wrapped Up

MAKES 4 SERVINGS

After years of packing sandwiches for her daughter's school lunch box, Janice got sick of making the same old turkey and cheese on whole wheat. To shake things up a bit without rocking the boat with daughter Carolyn, Janice created some fun and delicious alternatives. Turkey All Wrapped Up was Carolyn's hands-down favorite.

Moms Make It Over By . . .

- Adding avocado and salsa for vitamins, minerals, phytonutrients, and fiber.
- Switching to roasted turkey and reduced-fat cheese to lower the saturated fat, calories, and sodium.
- Using whole wheat flour tortillas for added nutrients and fiber.

6 ounces thinly sliced roasted turkey

½ cup preshredded reduced-fat Mexican blend or Cheddar cheese

¼ cup salsa

½ ripe avocado, peeled, pitted, and cut into thin slices

Four 8-inch whole wheat flour tortillas

1. Arrange the turkey, cheese, salsa, and avocado down the center of each of the tortillas.

2. Roll up tightly and slice in half.

PREPARATION TIME: 10 MINUTES

Moms' Kitchen Notes: To keep the avocado from turning brown in a lunch box, wrap the sandwich tightly in plastic wrap.

	Before	After
Calories	380	190
Fat (g)	21	7
Saturated Fat (g)	7	2
Sodium (mg)	1,450	690
Carbohydrate (g)	29	26
Fiber (g)	1	3
Protein (g)	19	15

The Full Monte Cristo

MAKES 4 SERVINGS

When is a ham and cheese sandwich more than a ham and cheese sandwich? The answer: When it's a Monte Cristo. This old-fashioned ham, cheese, and turkey sandwich is dipped in an egg batter, fried in butter, and served with jelly and powdered sugar. We really loved the original flavor, but all the saturated fat and calories were a big turnoff.

Moms Make It Over By . . .

- Switching to a smaller portion of reduced-fat cheese and lean deli ham, and cooking in a moderate amount of healthy canola oil to lower the saturated fat, calories, and sodium.
- Using whole wheat bread for added nutrients and fiber.

¼ cup all-fruit apricot jam

8 slices 100% whole wheat bread

3 ounces thinly sliced lean deli ham

3 ounces thinly sliced reduced-fat Provolone or Swiss cheese

4 teaspoons honey mustard

3 large eggs

3 tablespoons 1% lowfat milk

1 tablespoon canola oil

1. Spread 1 tablespoon jam over each of 4 bread slices. Top each evenly with the ham and cheese.

2. Spread 1 teaspoon mustard on each of the 4 remaining bread slices. Place firmly on the ham and cheese. Set aside.

3. Whisk together the eggs and milk in a large bowl. Dip the sandwiches in the egg mixture, turning carefully to coat.

4. Heat half the oil in a large nonstick skillet over medium-high heat. Add the sandwiches and cook until the bottoms are golden brown, 3 to 4 minutes.

5. Add the remaining oil, flip the sandwiches, and cook until the bottoms are golden brown and the cheese melts, an additional 3 to 4 minutes. Slice and serve warm.

PREPARATION TIME: 15 MINUTES
COOKING TIME: 10 MINUTES

Moms' Kitchen Notes: Serve with sliced kiwi or mango.

	Before	After
Calories	570	380
Fat (g)	29	16
Saturated Fat (g)	15	5
Sodium (mg)	1,210	660
Carbohydrate (g)	48	43
Fiber (g)	1	4
Protein (g)	27	22

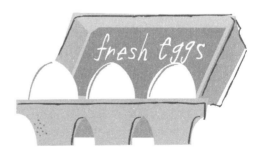

CHAPTER 7

Breakfast for Dinner

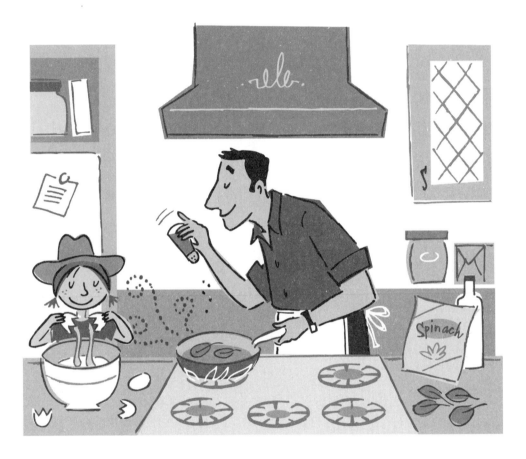

Broccoli Quiche Lorraine • Quick Corn & Ham Pudding • Cowboy Breakfast Wraps • Blueberry Banana Pancakes • Hearty Cornmeal Apple Pancakes • Pastina with Peas • Corned Beef & Carrot Hash • Sweet Potato Walnut Waffles • Potato Olé Omelet • Fruity French Toast • Super Sausage & Broccoli Strata • Berry Best Blintzes

Have you ever had one of those nights where the only meal you could muster up was a bowl of cereal? The children don't usually mind because, after all, breakfast tends to be their favorite meal of the day. But making a meal out of Cocoa Puffs or Frosted Flakes may leave the kids feeling pretty hungry a few short hours later. Thankfully, plenty of other breakfast options are just as easy to prepare (well, almost) when you're in a pinch.

Most of our breakfast entrées have one thing in common: eggs. Now just in case you're sitting there thinking, "Are you guys crazy? Eggs can't possibly be good for my family," consider the latest dietary guidelines from the American Heart Association that permit eating up to one egg a day, or seven a week, as long as it's part of an overall heart-healthy diet.

We think eggs are awesome. Sure, eggs contain cholesterol, but they're surprisingly low in saturated fat, one of the real culprits in heart disease. In fact, eggs contain slightly more heart-healthy monounsaturated fats (1.91 grams/egg) than saturated fat (1.55 grams/egg). They're a convenient, inexpensive, and low-calorie source of high-quality protein and come packaged with important vitamins and minerals, including vitamin A, vitamin E, iron, zinc, and folate . . . a B vitamin that can actually help to reduce the risk of heart disease. Bear in mind too that most of the nutrients in eggs are found in the yolk so if you've been washing them down the drain, we hope you'll come to enjoy eating the entire egg once again without guilt.

Okay. So eggs are off the hook (especially when you buy omega-3 eggs). But we can't ignore the fact that when eggs are on the menu, they're often accompanied by greasy sausages, bacon, butter, and hash browns. Those mealtime accomplices—loaded with saturated fat and sodium—deserve the bad rap, not the eggs.

Our recipe makeovers focus on everything from slashing the saturated fat to boosting the fiber. Perhaps the most dramatic is our remake of the classic quiche Lorraine, where we manage to remove nearly 40 grams of saturated fat and 700 calories from each serving alone. That's a tough act to follow, but as you read on, you'll discover a dozen new ways to enjoy quick, super-nourishing breakfast favorites . . . even when it's dinnertime.

Broccoli Quiche Lorraine

MAKES 4 SERVINGS

When we sat down to discuss quiche Lorraine, we concluded that it needed more than a makeover . . . it needed a complete overhaul. Traditionally made with a flaky, rich pie crust, heavy whipping cream, and ¼ pound of bacon, we knew we could work wonders with this recipe . . . and we did.

Moms Make It Over By . . .

- Adding broccoli for vitamins, minerals, phytonutrients, and fiber.
- Using reduced-fat cheese, lowfat milk, lean deli ham, and going "crustless" to slash the saturated fat and calories.
- Using less added salt and eliminating the bacon to reduce the sodium.

> 2 cups fresh or frozen broccoli
>
> 2 tablespoons dried bread crumbs
>
> 2 ounces lean deli ham, diced
>
> 1 cup preshredded reduced-fat Cheddar cheese
>
> 5 large eggs
>
> 1 cup 1% lowfat milk
>
> ¼ teaspoon salt
>
> ⅛ teaspoon dried thyme or ½ teaspoon fresh thyme
>
> Pinch of pepper
>
> ¼ cup grated Parmesan cheese

1. Steam the broccoli until tender, about 5 minutes. Coarsely chop and set aside.

2. Preheat the oven to 375°F.

3. Lightly oil or coat a 9-inch pie plate with nonstick cooking spray. Sprinkle the bottom and sides with the bread crumbs. Arrange the broccoli, ham, and Cheddar cheese over the bottom of the pie plate.

4. Whisk together the eggs, milk, salt, thyme, and pepper in a medium bowl.

5. Pour the egg mixture over the broccoli and top with the Parmesan cheese.

6. Bake uncovered until golden brown, 35 to 40 minutes.

PREPARATION TIME: 15 MINUTES
COOKING TIME: 35 TO 40 MINUTES

	Before	After
Calories	980	280
Fat (g)	80	15
Saturated Fat (g)	44	7
Sodium (mg)	1,260	540
Carbohydrate (g)	51	11
Fiber (g)	2	2
Protein (g)	14	26

Moms' Kitchen Notes: For this recipe, Liz prefers thinly sliced deli ham, while Janice likes a thicker cut. The choice is yours.

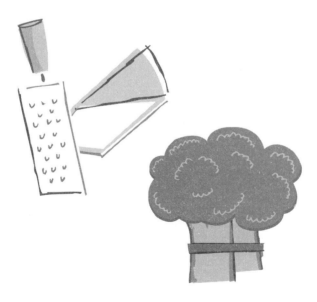

The Hen That Laid the Omega-3 Egg

What do eggs and salmon have in common? Not too much, unless of course you buy a "designer egg" rich in omega-3 fatty acids. Omega-3 fats, the type found in cold-water fish such as salmon and mackerel, have powerful health benefits, including reducing the risk of heart attacks and high blood pressure. New research shows they may also help to alleviate the symptoms of rheumatoid arthritis and depression.

So how does a fatty acid found in fish find its way into an egg? The answer is in the feed. Chickens that lay omega-3 eggs are fed a special diet rich in things like flaxseed, fish oil, and sea algae. The result is an egg with anywhere from 100 to 200 milligrams of omega-3s but no fishy taste! To put those numbers in perspective, you would have to eat about a dozen omega-3 eggs to equal the amount of omega-3 fatty acids found in 3 ounces of salmon. But the way we look at it, every little bit counts. As for the cost, it's about 10 cents more per egg . . . a cost we believe is well worth it, given the health benefits. Most supermarkets now carry omega-3 eggs. Look for them next to the regular eggs or in the health food section.

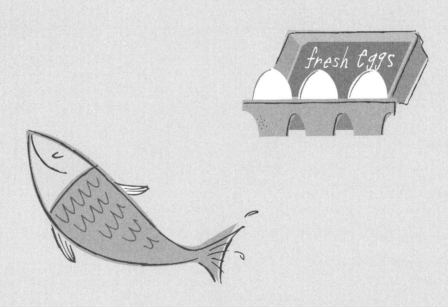

Quick Corn & Ham Pudding

MAKES 4 TO 6 SERVINGS

When your finicky eater gobbles up a dish at a friend's house, your first question should be: "Can I have that recipe?" That's exactly what Janice did when her daughter Carolyn tried this rich and creamy corn pudding. With a few small adjustments to the recipe, it's now a healthy quichelike dinner staple at the Bissex house.

Moms Make It Over By . . .

🍓 Using lowfat milk, reduced-fat cheese, and lean deli ham to lower the saturated fat and calories.

1½ cups 1% lowfat milk

¼ cup all-purpose flour

5 large eggs, beaten

2 cups frozen corn kernels, thawed

4 ounces lean deli ham, finely diced

4 ounces reduced-fat Swiss cheese, finely diced

¼ cup grated Parmesan cheese

1. Preheat the oven to 375°F.

2. Lightly oil or coat a 7 x 11-inch baking pan with nonstick cooking spray and set aside.

3. Whisk together the milk and flour in a large bowl until well blended. Add the eggs, corn, ham, Swiss cheese, and Parmesan cheese, and whisk to combine.

4. Pour the mixture into the prepared pan and bake, uncovered, until golden brown, about 40 minutes.

PREPARATION TIME: 10 MINUTES
COOKING TIME: 40 MINUTES

	Before	After
Calories	500	340
Fat (g)	41	15
Saturated Fat (g)	23	7
Sodium (mg)	660	580
Carbohydrate (g)	17	26
Fiber (g)	2	2
Protein (g)	17	26

Moms' Kitchen Notes: Serve with grilled or steamed asparagus and a warm whole grain roll.

Cowboy Breakfast Wraps

MAKES 4 SERVINGS

When we think of huevos rancheros—a hearty breakfast dish of fried eggs, sausage, salsa, and tortillas—we think of cowboys riding on the open range, rustling up cattle, and eating by the campfire at night. All those images of the wild wild West inspired us to come up with our own version of huevos rancheros. But in place of fried sausages, we turned to spinach instead. In the end, we stoked up the nutritional profile of the meal while still pleasing our kids.

Moms Make It Over By . . .

🍓 Adding spinach for vitamins, minerals, phytonutrients, and fiber.

🍓 Eliminating the sausage to lower the saturated fat, sodium, and calories.

> 1 tablespoon olive oil
>
> One 6-ounce bag prewashed baby spinach (about 4 packed cups)
>
> Pinch of kosher salt
>
> 5 large eggs, beaten
>
> ½ cup preshredded reduced-fat Cheddar cheese
>
> Four 8-inch flour tortillas
>
> ¼ to ½ cup mild salsa

1. Heat the oil in a large nonstick skillet over medium-high heat. Add the spinach and cook, stirring occasionally, until the spinach wilts, 3 to 5 minutes. Season with salt.

2. Add the eggs and cheese and cook, stirring frequently, until the eggs are set, about 2 minutes.

3. Stack the tortillas on a microwave-safe plate, uncovered, and heat in the microwave until warmed through, 30 to 45 seconds.

4. Assemble the wraps by placing a quarter of the egg mixture down the center of each tortilla. Top with 1 to 2 tablespoons of salsa and wrap burrito-style.

PREPARATION TIME: 5 MINUTES
COOKING TIME: 10 MINUTES

Moms' Kitchen Notes: Serve with sliced melon or grapes.

	Before	After
Calories	530	320
Fat (g)	40	14
Saturated Fat (g)	14	3
Sodium (mg)	1,150	560
Carbohydrate (g)	18	30
Fiber (g)	3	4
Protein (g)	26	16

Blueberry Banana Pancakes

MAKES ABOUT FIFTEEN 4-INCH PANCAKES, 4 TO 5 SERVINGS

If the sight of pancakes whets your appetite for gobs of whipped butter, sweet syrup, and savory sausages, we hope our pancake makeover will be just as tempting. These fruit-filled pancakes are a staple at Liz's house where all her boys, even hubby Tim, ask for them weekly.

Moms Make It Over By . . .

- Adding blueberries, banana, and wheat germ for vitamins, minerals, phytonutrients, and fiber.
- Cooking in a moderate amount of healthy canola oil versus butter to lower the saturated fat.

    1½ cups all-purpose flour

    ⅓ cup wheat germ

    ⅓ cup quick-cooking oats

    1 tablespoon baking powder

    ½ teaspoon ground cinnamon

    ⅛ teaspoon salt

    2 large eggs, beaten

    1½ cups 1% lowfat milk

    1 ripe banana, mashed (about ½ cup)

    2 tablespoons pure maple syrup

    4 teaspoons canola oil

    1 cup frozen or fresh blueberries

1. Whisk together the flour, wheat germ, oats, baking powder, cinnamon, and salt in a large bowl until well combined. Set aside.

2. Whisk together the eggs, milk, banana, and maple syrup in a medium bowl until blended.

3. Pour the liquid ingredients over the dry ingredients and stir until just moistened.

4. Meanwhile, heat 1 teaspoon of the oil in a large nonstick skillet or griddle over medium-high heat.

5. Pour the batter onto the hot skillet or griddle, using a ¼-cup measuring cup, forming 4-inch cakes. Using a spoon (so your fingers don't turn blue), arrange the blueberries evenly on each pancake. Adjust the heat if the skillet gets too hot.

6. Cook until bubbles begin to appear on the surface of the pancakes and the bottoms turn golden brown, 2 to 3 minutes. Flip and cook until golden brown, an additional 2 to 3 minutes.

7. Repeat with the remaining oil, batter, and blueberries.

PREPARATION TIME: 10 MINUTES
COOKING TIME: 20 MINUTES

	Before	After
Calories	410	380
Fat (g)	18	9
Saturated Fat (g)	8	2
Sodium (mg)	640	460
Carbohydrate (g)	50	61
Fiber (g)	1	4
Protein (g)	11	14

Moms' Kitchen Notes: Top with pure maple syrup and serve with light breakfast sausage.

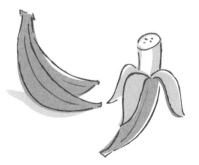

Hearty Cornmeal Apple Pancakes

MAKES ABOUT FIFTEEN 4-INCH PANCAKES, 5 SERVINGS

When Janice was growing up, her dad made pancakes every Sunday morning for breakfast. His recipe called for flour, milk, eggs, and butter. Today, Janice keeps the family tradition alive with a heartier version perfect for lazy weekends as well as hectic weeknights.

Moms Make It Over By . . .

- Adding apple for vitamins, phytonutrients, and fiber.
- Using whole wheat flour, cornmeal, and wheat germ for added nutrients and fiber.

    2 large eggs

    1¾ cups 1% lowfat milk

    ⅔ cup all-purpose flour

    ⅔ cup whole wheat flour

    ⅔ cup cornmeal

    ⅓ cup wheat germ

    ⅓ cup sugar

    1 tablespoon baking powder

    ½ teaspoon salt

    1 large apple, peeled, cored, and finely chopped

    4 teaspoons canola oil

    ¼ cup pecans, chopped, optional

    ¼ cup mini chocolate chips, optional

1. Whisk together the eggs and milk in a medium bowl. Set aside.

2. Whisk together the all-purpose flour, whole wheat flour, cornmeal, wheat germ, sugar, baking powder, and salt in a large bowl until well combined.

3. Pour the liquid ingredients over the dry ingredients and stir until blended. Add the apple and stir to combine.

4. Heat 1 teaspoon of the oil in a large, nonstick skillet or griddle over medium-high heat.

5. Pour the pancake batter onto the hot skillet or griddle, using a ¼-cup measuring cup, forming 4-inch cakes. Top with the optional ingredients if desired. Adjust the heat if the skillet gets too hot.

6. Cook until bubbles begin to appear on the surface of the pancakes and the bottoms turn golden brown, 2 to 3 minutes. Flip and cook until golden brown, an additional 2 minutes.

7. Repeat with the remaining oil, batter, and optional ingredients.

PREPARATION TIME: 10 MINUTES
COOKING TIME: 20 MINUTES

	Before	After
Calories	410	370
Fat (g)	18	9
Saturated Fat (g)	8	2
Sodium (mg)	640	570
Carbohydrate (g)	50	63
Fiber (g)	1	5
Protein (g)	11	13

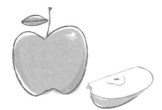

Pastina with Peas

MAKES 4 SERVINGS

It's funny how when friends hear you're writing a cookbook, they start leaving recipes in your mailbox! The original recipe for pastina came from the mother of a one-year-old, who calls her simple dish of pasta, eggs, and butter "comfort food for a toddler's soul." She wanted to know how to make it more nutritious, so we showed her how.

Moms Make It Over By . . .

- Adding peas for vitamins, minerals, phytonutrients, and fiber.
- Eliminating the butter to lower the saturated fat and calories.

    2 cups all-natural chicken broth or vegetable broth

    1 cup water

    6 ounces pastina (about ¾ cup) or other small dried pasta such as alphabets or orzo

    1½ cups frozen peas

    ¼ teaspoon onion powder

    3 large eggs, beaten

    ⅓ cup grated Parmesan cheese

1. Combine the broth, water, pasta, peas, and onion powder in a medium saucepan. Place over high heat and bring to a boil. Reduce the heat and cook at a low boil until the pasta is tender, about 5 minutes. Do not drain.

2. Add the eggs and Parmesan cheese and cook, stirring constantly, until the eggs are set, 2 to 4 minutes.

3. Serve in individual bowls.

PREPARATION TIME: 5 MINUTES
COOKING TIME: 10 MINUTES

	Before	After
Calories	380	280
Fat (g)	20	7
Saturated Fat (g)	11	2.5
Sodium (mg)	660	500
Carbohydrate (g)	33	40
Fiber (g)	1	4
Protein (g)	16	13

Be Egg-stra Careful

Ordering your eggs sunny side up or soft-boiled is now considered a food safety faux pas. The reason: Eating undercooked eggs can put you at risk for salmonella food poisoning. While only about 1 in 20,000 eggs may contain this dangerous bacterium, it's a risk worth noting given the fact that in the United States alone, over 5 billion dozen eggs are produced each year.

The following food safety dos and don'ts should keep you and your family safer when eggs are on the menu:

- DO wash your hands and all utensils with hot soapy water after touching raw eggs.
- DON'T store your eggs in the refrigerator door because the temperature there can rise above 40°F, allowing bacteria to grow.
- DO cook egg dishes to 160°F.
- DON'T wash eggs before you store them because it removes their protective coating.
- DO throw cracked eggs away.
- DON'T eat yolks that are runny.

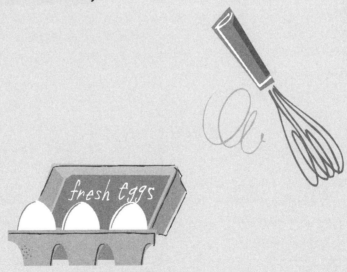

Corned Beef & Carrot Hash

MAKES 4 SERVINGS

Corned beef hash is an old stick-to-your-ribs (and waistline) favorite that we easily updated with good nutrition in mind. With the help of lean deli corned beef and a few cups of carrots, we managed to deep-six much of the saturated fat and sodium while increasing the vitamin A tenfold.

Moms Make It Over By . . .

- 🥕 Adding carrots for vitamins, minerals, phytonutrients, and fiber.
- 🥕 Using lean deli corned beef and using lowfat milk in the white sauce to lower the saturated fat, sodium, and calories.

1 tablespoon olive oil

3 cups frozen shredded hash brown potatoes

One 10-ounce bag preshredded carrots, or 3 large carrots, shredded (about 3 cups)

8 ounces lean deli corned beef, diced

1 teaspoon onion powder

½ teaspoon garlic powder

¼ teaspoon salt

Pinch of pepper

1 cup 1% lowfat milk or 1 cup all-natural chicken broth

1 tablespoon all-purpose flour

1. Heat the oil in a large nonstick skillet over medium-high heat. Add the potatoes, carrots, corned beef, onion powder, garlic powder, salt, and pepper. Cook, stirring frequently, until the potatoes and carrots are tender, about 10 minutes.

2. Meanwhile, whisk together the milk and flour in a medium bowl until well blended.

3. Pour the milk mixture into the skillet and stir until heated through and thickened, about 2 minutes.

PREPARATION TIME: 10 MINUTES
COOKING TIME: 15 MINUTES

Moms' Kitchen Notes: A scrambled or fried egg (in olive oil of course) is a nice addition to the meal, along with sliced melon.

	Before	After
Calories	620	220
Fat (g)	36	6
Saturated Fat (g)	12	1.5
Sodium (mg)	1,830	690
Carbohydrate (g)	21	30
Fiber (g)	2	4
Protein (g)	51	16

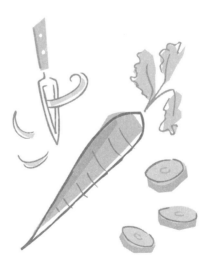

Sweet Potato Walnut Waffles

MAKES EIGHT 4-INCH SQUARE WAFFLES, 4 SERVINGS

If waffles and whipped cream go hand in hand at your house, try waffles and sweet potatoes instead. If you think we're adding sweet potatoes for the sake of more nutrients and fiber, you're right. But you'll also be pleasantly surprised when you taste them. Flavor is number one! If you don't have a waffle iron, maybe it's time to add it to your holiday wish list.

Moms Make It Over By . . .

- Adding sweet potatoes for vitamins, minerals, phytonutrients, and fiber.
- Using a moderate amount of healthy canola oil versus a lot of butter to lower the saturated fat and calories.
- Using whole wheat flour for added nutrients and fiber.
- Including walnuts for added nutrients and healthy omega-3 fats.

3 large eggs, beaten

1½ cups 1% lowfat milk

One-half of a 15¾-ounce can sweet potatoes, drained and mashed (about ½ cup)

1 tablespoon canola oil

1 teaspoon vanilla extract

1 cup all-purpose flour

½ cup whole wheat flour

½ cup walnuts, finely chopped

2 teaspoons baking powder

¾ teaspoon ground cinnamon

¼ teaspoon salt

Pure maple syrup

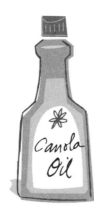

1. Preheat the waffle iron according to the manufacturer's instructions.

2. Whisk together the eggs and milk in a medium bowl. Add the sweet potatoes, canola oil, and vanilla and stir to combine.

3. Combine the all-purpose flour, whole wheat flour, walnuts, baking powder, cinnamon, and salt in a large bowl.

4. Add the egg mixture to the dry ingredients and stir until just moistened.

5. Coat the hot waffle iron with nonstick cooking spray. Pour the batter onto the hot waffle iron, to cover about two-thirds of the grid surface. Cook according to the manufacturer's instructions. The waffles may need to cook for an additional minute due to the added sweet potatoes. Repeat with the remaining batter.

6. Serve hot with pure maple syrup.

PREPARATION TIME: 15 MINUTES
COOKING TIME: 15 MINUTES

	Before	After
Calories	580	460
Fat (g)	36	19
Saturated Fat (g)	21	3
Sodium (mg)	750	500
Carbohydrate (g)	51	56
Fiber (g)	1	5
Protein (g)	14	16

Moms' Kitchen Notes: For banana waffles, mash one ripe banana and add it to the batter in place of the sweet potatoes. Freeze leftover sweet potatoes in a resealable plastic bag for later use.

Potato Olé Omelet

MAKES 4 SERVINGS

We love olive oil, but when a recipe calls for more than ½ cup, we have to draw the line. That was the case with the traditional Spanish omelet Janice learned to make during one college semester in Spain. With some trial and error in the kitchen, she discovered a new way to keep the rich Mediterranean flavors with a more reasonable amount of healthy fat. Top with a tablespoon of ketchup for an extra kid-friendly kick.

Moms Make It Over By ...

- Adding bell peppers for vitamins, minerals, phytonutrients, and fiber.
- Using a moderate amount of healthy olive oil to lower the calories.

> 2 tablespoons olive oil
>
> 2 cups frozen shredded hash brown potatoes
>
> 2 cups frozen mixed bell pepper strips or 1 medium red bell pepper, finely diced (about 1 cup)
>
> 1 teaspoon onion powder
>
> ½ teaspoon garlic powder
>
> ½ teaspoon salt
>
> 6 large eggs
>
> ¼ cup 1% lowfat milk

1. Heat 1 tablespoon of the oil in a large nonstick skillet over medium-high heat.

2. Add the potatoes, bell peppers, onion powder, garlic powder, and salt and cook, stirring frequently, until the vegetables are tender, about 6 minutes.

3. Meanwhile, whisk together the eggs and milk in a large bowl. Add the cooked vegetables and stir to combine.

4. Heat the remaining oil in the skillet over medium-high heat. Pour the egg mixture back into the skillet, reduce the heat to medium, and cook until the omelet turns golden brown on the bottom, 3 to 5 minutes.

5. Preheat the broiler.

6. Place the skillet under the broiler. If the handle is plastic, wrap it in aluminum foil or slide the omelet carefully onto a large baking sheet. Broil until the top turns golden brown, 3 to 5 minutes.

7. Cut into wedges and serve.

PREPARATION TIME: 10 MINUTES
COOKING TIME: 15 MINUTES

	Before	After
Calories	530	250
Fat (g)	42	16
Saturated Fat (g)	7	3.5
Sodium (mg)	680	410
Carbohydrate (g)	28	16
Fiber (g)	2	2
Protein (g)	12	12

Moms' Kitchen Notes: If your kids don't like bell peppers, use 2 cups frozen mixed vegetables instead.

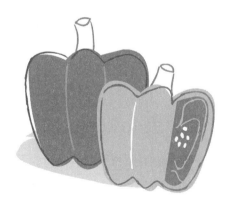

Fruity French Toast

MAKES 4 SERVINGS

For many busy moms, the ultimate last-minute meal is French toast. Hey, the ingredients couldn't be more basic: slices of Wonder Bread, eggs, and some milk. Our new-and-improved recipe is just as basic (minus the white bread, of course), and you'll love our creative new topping.

Moms Make It Over By . . .

- ✿ Adding pears and raisins for vitamins, minerals, phytonutrients, and fiber.
- ✿ Using whole wheat bread for added nutrients and fiber.
- ✿ Cooking in a moderate amount of healthy canola oil versus butter to lower the saturated fat.

> **One 15-ounce can unsweetened pear halves**
>
> **2 teaspoons cornstarch**
>
> **¼ teaspoon ground cinnamon**
>
> **¼ cup golden raisins**
>
> **¼ cup walnuts or pecans, coarsely chopped, optional**
>
> **4 large eggs**
>
> **2 tablespoons 1% lowfat milk**
>
> **2 tablespoons apple juice**
>
> **½ teaspoon ground cinnamon**
>
> **¼ teaspoon vanilla extract**
>
> **1 tablespoon canola oil**
>
> **8 slices 100% whole wheat bread**

1. Drain the pear halves and reserve the liquid. Slice the pears into quarters and set aside.

2. Combine the reserved pear liquid, cornstarch, and cinnamon in a small saucepan and whisk until well blended.

3. Place the saucepan over medium-high heat. Add the raisins and bring to a simmer, stirring constantly. Reduce the heat and continue to simmer and stir gently until the mixture thickens slightly, about 2 minutes. Add the pears and the nuts, if desired. Stir and warm through. Set aside, covered, until the French toast is cooked.

4. Meanwhile, whisk together the eggs, milk, apple juice, cinnamon, and vanilla in a large bowl.

5. Heat half the oil in a large nonstick skillet over medium-high heat.

6. Dip the bread in the egg mixture, one slice at a time, and coat evenly. Place the bread in the skillet and cook until the bottoms turn golden brown, 2 to 3 minutes per side.

7. Remove to a plate, cover, and set aside. Repeat with the remaining oil and bread slices. Serve with the pear topping.

PREPARATION TIME: 15 MINUTES
COOKING TIME: 15 MINUTES

Moms' Kitchen Notes: Serve with an orange juice spritzer made with equal parts orange juice and seltzer water.

	Before	After
Calories	410	350
Fat (g)	23	11
Saturated Fat (g)	11	2.5
Sodium (mg)	640	370
Carbohydrate (g)	36	54
Fiber (g)	1	6
Protein (g)	14	12

Super Sausage & Broccoli Strata

MAKES 6 SERVINGS

Where there's a will there's a way. That was precisely our attitude when we gave the classic cheese strata—initially made with white bread, whole milk, sausage, and full-fat cheese— a makeover. We discovered some convenient ways to slash the bad fat while sneaking in the good nutrition.

Moms Make It Over By . . .

- Adding broccoli for vitamins, minerals, phytonutrients, and fiber.
- Using whole grain bread for added nutrients and fiber.
- Using lowfat milk and light sausage to lower the saturated fat, sodium, and calories.

One 10-ounce box frozen chopped broccoli

5 large eggs

1½ cups 1% lowfat milk

1 tablespoon Dijon mustard

¼ teaspoon salt

7 cups (about 7 slices) multigrain or 100% whole wheat bread cut into ½-inch cubes

One 8-ounce package frozen, precooked light breakfast sausage, thawed and thinly sliced

1 cup preshredded reduced-fat Cheddar cheese, divided

1. Lightly oil or coat a 7 x 11-inch baking pan with nonstick cooking spray and set aside.

2. Steam the broccoli until tender, about 5 minutes.

3. Whisk together the eggs, milk, mustard, and salt in a large bowl until well blended. Add the bread, sausage, and broccoli and toss to coat evenly. Set aside for 10 minutes.

4. Preheat the oven to 375°F.

5. Place half the bread mixture in the baking pan, sprinkle with half the cheese, and then top with the remaining bread mixture.

6. Bake uncovered 30 minutes, sprinkle with the remaining cheese, and bake until the cheese melts, an additional 5 minutes. Let stand 5 minutes, cut into squares, and serve.

PREPARATION TIME: 15 MINUTES
COOKING TIME: 40 MINUTES

Moms' Kitchen Notes: To use fresh broccoli, steam 3 or 4 cups and then coarsely chop.

	Before	After
Calories	700	300
Fat (g)	42	15
Saturated Fat (g)	18	5
Sodium (mg)	1,500	730
Carbohydrate (g)	40	22
Fiber (g)	2	4
Protein (g)	38	22

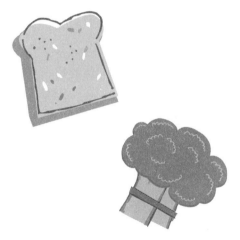

Berry Best Blintzes

MAKES 3 SERVINGS

If you've ever gone to the trouble of making cheese blintzes from scratch you may never do it again once you try frozen blintzes. We love them because many brands are surprisingly low in saturated fat and also taste great. With our simple berry topping, they're a Meal Makeover Mom's delight.

Moms Make It Over By . . .

- Adding blueberries and strawberries for vitamins, minerals, phytonutrients, and fiber.
- Using a lower-fat frozen blintz to lower the saturated fat and calories.

> One 13-ounce package frozen cheese blintzes
>
> 2 tablespoons all-fruit strawberry jam
>
> 1½ cups sliced fresh strawberries
>
> 1 cup fresh or frozen blueberries
>
> ½ to 1 cup lowfat vanilla yogurt

1. Cook the blintzes according to package directions.

2. To make the topping, heat the jam in a medium saucepan over medium heat, stirring until melted. Add the strawberries and blueberries, stir to coat, and cook until heated through, about 3 minutes. Remove from the heat.

3. Serve the blintzes on individual plates and top with the berries and yogurt.

PREPARATION TIME: 10 MINUTES
COOKING TIME: 10 TO 20 MINUTES

	Before	After
Calories	530	280
Fat (g)	33	5
Saturated Fat (g)	17	1.5
Sodium (mg)	840	300
Carbohydrate (g)	36	52
Fiber (g)	<1	7
Protein (g)	21	15

Moms' Kitchen Notes: Serve with light breakfast sausage.

CHAPTER 8

Pasta & Pizza Perfection

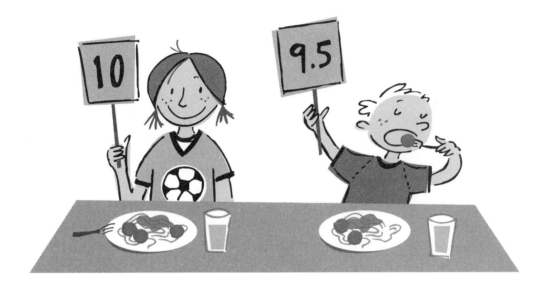

Fast-As-Boxed Macaroni & Cheese • Mama's Amazing Ziti • Cheese Ravioli with Pumpkin Sauce • Sweet & Nutty Thai Thing • Tortellini with Broccoli "Pesto" • Squishy Squash Lasagna • Wagon Wheel Alfredo • Kitchen Sink Pasta Salad • Eggplant Parm in a Pot • Thai Chicken Pizza • Cheeseburger Pizza • Pizza Bonita

Where would we be without macaroni & cheese? For that matter, where would we be without spaghetti, ravioli, tortellini, and the dozens of other pasta shapes and varieties that we've come to rely on as dinner staples? We can all thank our third president, Thomas Jefferson, for helping to introduce pasta to America. During his presidency, he had it shipped in from Italy and was even known to serve dishes like macaroni & cheese at the White House. Hey, maybe it was a delicacy back then.

Of course, if you fast-forward to today, pasta is more than a novelty, it's a necessity. Although Italians still eat more pasta than anyone else on the planet, Americans manage to devour over 20 pounds per person each year. It's no wonder. Pasta is versatile, easy, and fast, not to mention fun and delicious. It's also nutritious. A ½-cup serving has less than 100 calories and a minimal amount of fat *and* is a good source of B vitamins, folic acid, and iron. With such stellar credentials, why then has pasta gotten such a bad rap over the years? Well, we think it's because many Americans often fill up on heaping platefuls of the stuff, smothering it with heavy cream sauces and butter. Look at fettuccine Alfredo, for example. A typical serving has over 900 calories and 50 grams of fat! The bottom line: If you eat too much of anything, whether it's pasta, bread, beef, or bananas, you can say *arrivederci* to your waistline.

Now, speaking of fettuccine Alfredo, you'll say bravo when you see how we rescued the traditional recipe. Instead of the usual cup of heavy cream and boatloads of butter, we created a leaner cheese sauce that brought the fat down to a more respectable 11 grams. We even tossed in some sweet little green peas to boost the goodness of this dish. Our macaroni & cheese makeover, which we must admit was pretty clever, illustrates how easy it can be to make from scratch. Our recipe uses "real" ingredients and takes about the same few minutes to prepare as the mac & cheese from a box. It's also a whole lot healthier with double the calcium and half the fat.

And then, of course, there's pizza, another family favorite. Pizza is so popular, in fact, that every year Americans eat a staggering three billion pies. But pizza often delivers more saturated fat and calories than you'd expect. Sit down to two slices of your basic cheese pizza and you get about 500 calories, 14 grams of fat (about half of them saturated), and 880 milligrams of sodium. Not too bad. But order a pizza with sausage and pepperoni and you're talking close to 1,000 calories, 50 grams of fat, and over 2,000 milligrams of sodium in two slices alone. We have a solution: Make your pizzas at home. In the time it takes to pick up the phone, order a pizza, and wait for the delivery guy to arrive, you can create your own. So for a pizza and pasta renovation, read on!

Pasta Particulars

Wondering why your pasta often comes out mushy, sticks together, or yields more than your family of four could possibly eat in a meal? Read our pointers and find your answers.

- To cook perfect pasta every time, boil 4 to 6 quarts of water for every pound of pasta. Use a generous amount of water and follow the suggested cooking times to prevent pasta from sticking together or turning into a big gooey glob.
- Pasta is considered cooked when it is "al dente," which means it's firm to the bite yet cooked through.
- When you drain your pasta, reserve some of the cooking water. The water, which contains starch from the noodles, can help to moisten the pasta and thicken the sauce when a small amount is added back to the dish.
- The suggested serving size for pasta is 2 ounces uncooked (about ½ cup). Therefore, a 16-ounce box of pasta (aka 1 pound) should feed about 8 people. Bear in mind that a toddler may end up eating barely 1 ounce while Mom or Dad may eat 3. So the 2-ounce guideline is flexible.
- Two ounces of uncooked pasta yields about 1 cup cooked.
- Whole wheat pasta is a healthy alternative to regular pasta. In fact, a 2-ounce portion of whole wheat pasta has about 6 grams of fiber compared to 2 grams in regular pasta. You can use whole wheat pasta in any recipe that calls for pasta.

Fast-As-Boxed Macaroni & Cheese

MAKES 4 SERVINGS

In 1936, Kraft Macaroni & Cheese was first introduced to U.S. consumers. Now, an astonishing one million boxes are sold each *day*. Mac & cheese from a box is an easy, kid-pleasing meal when you're in a pinch, but did you know it's just as fast (give or take a few minutes) to make it from scratch? Our homemade version may not have the same bright orange color as the stuff from a box, but kids love it and so will you . . . especially when you learn it has more calcium per serving than a glass of milk.

Moms Make It Over By . . .

 Using lowfat milk and reduced-fat cheese to increase the bone-building calcium and eliminating the butter to reduce the saturated fat and calories.

> 8 ounces dried small elbow macaroni (about 2 cups)
> 1½ cups 1% lowfat milk
> 2 tablespoons all-purpose flour
> 1 teaspoon Dijon mustard
> ½ teaspoon garlic powder
> 1½ cups preshredded reduced-fat Cheddar cheese
> 2 tablespoons grated Parmesan cheese

1. Cook the pasta according to package directions. Drain and set aside.

2. Return the saucepan to the stove (do not place over heat just yet). Add the milk, flour, mustard, and garlic powder and whisk until well blended.

3. Place over medium-high heat and bring to a simmer, stirring constantly. Reduce the heat and continue to simmer and stir gently until the mixture thickens slightly, about 2 minutes.

4. Add the Cheddar cheese and Parmesan cheese and stir until the cheese melts. Stir in the pasta, heat through, and serve.

PREPARATION TIME: 5 MINUTES
COOKING TIME: 15 MINUTES

Moms' Kitchen Notes: Add a 10-ounce package of your child's favorite frozen vegetable to the dish for a more complete meal. Just toss the veggies in with the pasta for the last 5 minutes of cooking.

	Before	After
Calories	410	340
Fat (g)	19	6
Saturated Fat (g)	5	3
Sodium (mg)	750	390
Carbohydrate (g)	49	48
Fiber (g)	1	2
Protein (g)	11	22

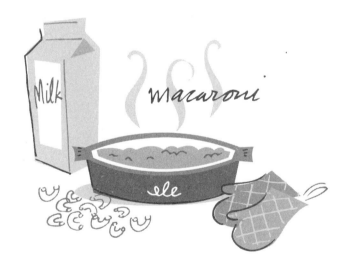

Mama's Amazing Ziti

MAKES 6 SERVINGS

When Liz was growing up, her mother's signature dish was an amazingly delicious baked ziti. Made with a pound of ground beef, half a pound of ziti, two cans of Campbell's Tomato Soup, and a ton of cheese, it was a big hit with the entire family. Even Liz's two sisters (perhaps the pickiest eaters of all time) ate it without complaint. Liz recently made an updated version of this unforgettable dish for her own family. While the memories came flooding back, much of the saturated fat and sodium became a thing of the past.

Moms Make It Over By . . .

- Adding carrots for vitamins, minerals, phytonutrients, and fiber.
- Switching to lean ground beef and part-skim cheese to lower the saturated fat and calories.
- Using reduced-sodium tomato soup to lower the sodium.

> 1 pound lean ground beef (90% or higher)
>
> 2 large carrots, shredded (about 2 cups), or 2 cups preshredded carrots
>
> Two 10¾-ounce cans 30%-less-sodium tomato soup
>
> 8 ounces dried ziti (about 2½ cups)
>
> 1 teaspoon dried basil
>
> ½ teaspoon garlic powder
>
> ½ teaspoon onion powder
>
> 1 cup preshredded part-skim mozzarella cheese
>
> ¼ cup grated Parmesan cheese

1. Place a large saucepan or Dutch oven over medium-high heat. Add the beef and carrots and cook, breaking up the large pieces, until the meat is no longer pink, about 5 minutes. Drain excess fat.

2. Add the tomato soup, 2 cans of water, ziti, basil, garlic powder, and onion powder and stir until well blended.

3. Bring the liquid to a boil, reduce the heat, and cook, covered, at a low boil, until the ziti is tender, about 25 minutes. Stir occasionally.

4. Stir in the mozzarella cheese. Serve in individual bowls and sprinkle with Parmesan cheese.

PREPARATION TIME: **10 MINUTES**
COOKING TIME: **30 MINUTES**

	Before	After
Calories	490	370
Fat (g)	23	9
Saturated Fat (g)	11	4.5
Sodium (mg)	800	580
Carbohydrate (g)	43	46
Fiber (g)	2	3
Protein (g)	28	27

Moms' Kitchen Notes: Serve with Simply Delicious Broccoli (page 318).

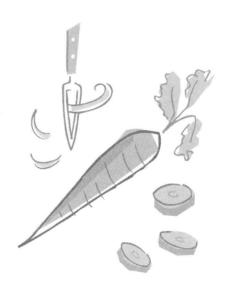

Cheese Ravioli with Pumpkin Sauce

MAKES 6 SERVINGS

How many times have your children requested ravioli with no sauce, just butter? We have nothing against a little bit of butter. In fact, we even use some in this antioxidant-packed Cheese Ravioli with Pumpkin Sauce. If you think we've gone way "out of the box" with this one, we have. But after trying it, we're confident you'll agree that pumpkin isn't just for pies anymore . . . it's for pasta, too.

Moms Make It Over By . . .

🍠 Adding pumpkin for vitamins, minerals, phytonutrients, and fiber.

🍠 Creating a sauce with pumpkin instead of all butter to lower the saturated fat and calories.

> One 15-ounce can 100% pure pumpkin
>
> 2 cups all-natural chicken broth or vegetable broth
>
> 3 tablespoons brown sugar
>
> 1 tablespoon butter
>
> ½ teaspoon garlic powder
>
> ½ teaspoon ground ginger or 1 teaspoon bottled minced ginger
>
> ½ teaspoon ground cinnamon
>
> ⅛ teaspoon ground nutmeg
>
> One 30-ounce bag frozen cheese ravioli
>
> ¼ cup reduced-fat sour cream, optional
>
> ¼ cup grated Parmesan cheese

1. Place a large saucepan of water over high heat. Cover and bring to a boil.

2. While the water is coming to a boil, combine the pumpkin, broth, sugar, butter, garlic powder, ginger, cinnamon, and nutmeg in a medium saucepan and stir to combine. Place over medium heat and bring to a simmer, stirring occasionally, until the butter melts and the mixture is heated through, about 10 minutes.

3. When the water comes to a boil, add the ravioli and cook according to package directions. Drain and set aside.

4. Just before serving, stir in the sour cream as desired. Serve the ravioli on individual plates, top with the pumpkin sauce, and sprinkle with Parmesan cheese.

PREPARATION TIME: 10 MINUTES
COOKING TIME: 10 MINUTES

	Before	After
Calories	420	370
Fat (g)	21	9
Saturated Fat (g)	13	5
Sodium (mg)	740	620
Carbohydrate (g)	37	49
Fiber (g)	1	4
Protein (g)	9	12

Moms' Kitchen Notes: When shopping for canned pumpkin, be careful not to pick up pumpkin pie mix by mistake!

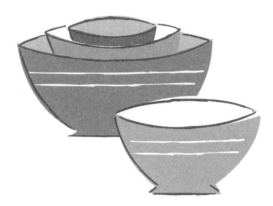

Sweet & Nutty Thai Thing

MAKES 4 TO 5 SERVINGS

One of our favorite Thai dishes is pad thai, traditionally made with exotic-sounding and sometimes hard to find ingredients like nam pla (Thai fish sauce), dried shrimp, and fresh chili peppers. It's not exactly the quickest thing to whip up when you're looking for a last-minute weeknight meal, so we simplified things a bit and came up with this kid-friendly Sweet & Nutty Thai Thing instead.

Moms Make It Over By . . .

🍓 Adding sweet potato for vitamins, minerals, phytonutrients, and fiber.

🍓 Using whole wheat pasta for added nutrients and fiber.

🍓 Eliminating the fish sauce to reduce the sodium.

🍓 Using about 2 ounces of dried pasta per serving to keep the portions and calories in check.

> 1 large sweet potato, peeled and cut into ½-inch cubes (about 3 cups)
>
> 8 ounces dried whole wheat rotini (about 3 cups)
>
> 1½ cups all-natural chicken broth
>
> 3 tablespoons all-purpose flour
>
> ¼ cup Thai peanut sauce or peanut satay stir-fry sauce
>
> ¾ teaspoon salt
>
> 8 ounces cooked skinless, boneless chicken breast halves, cut into bite-size pieces
>
> ¼ cup coarsely chopped dry roasted peanuts

1. Steam the sweet potato until tender, about 8 minutes. Set aside.

2. Cook the pasta according to package directions. Drain and set aside.

3. Return the saucepan to the stove (do not place over heat just yet). Add the broth, flour, peanut sauce, and salt and whisk until well blended.

4. Place over medium-high heat and bring to a simmer, stirring constantly. Reduce the heat and continue to simmer and stir gently until the mixture thickens slightly, about 2 minutes.

5. Stir in the pasta, sweet potato, and cooked chicken and heat through. Place in individual bowls, top with peanuts, and serve.

PREPARATION TIME: 15 MINUTES
COOKING TIME: 15 MINUTES

Moms' Kitchen Notes: For the cooked chicken in this dish, use leftovers or bake ½ pound skinless, boneless chicken breast halves at 350°F for about 20 minutes.

	Before	After
Calories	630	430
Fat (g)	34	8
Saturated Fat (g)	6	1.5
Sodium (mg)	1,630	660
Carbohydrate (g)	65	64
Fiber (g)	3	7
Protein (g)	29	27

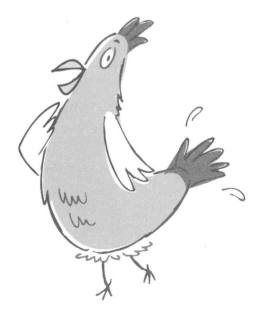

Tortellini with Broccoli "Pesto"

MAKES 4 SERVINGS

Pesto—that deliciously rich sauce of olive oil, pine nuts, Parmesan cheese, and basil—can transform a plain pasta dish into something spectacular. But if making it from scratch and having to use (and clean) your food processor on a busy weeknight is more than you can manage, try our very quick and very delicious compromise.

Moms Make It Over By . . .

- Adding broccoli for vitamins, minerals, phytonutrients, and fiber.
- Including walnuts for added nutrients and healthy omega-3 fats.

> One 12- or 16-ounce bag frozen cheese tortellini
>
> One 16-ounce bag frozen broccoli florets, or 1 head broccoli, cut into small florets (5 to 6 cups)
>
> ½ cup walnuts, toasted and coarsely chopped, or ¼ cup pine nuts, lightly toasted
>
> ¼ cup grated Parmesan cheese
>
> 2 tablespoons extra virgin olive oil
>
> ¼ teaspoon kosher salt
>
> ⅛ teaspoon garlic powder

1. Cook the tortellini in a large saucepan according to package directions. Five minutes before they're done, add the broccoli. Bring the water back to a boil and cook until the broccoli and tortellini are tender. Drain and return to the pan.

2. Immediately add the walnuts, Parmesan cheese, oil, salt, and garlic powder and stir well to combine.

PREPARATION TIME: 10 MINUTES
COOKING TIME: 10 MINUTES

	Before	After
Calories	570	480
Fat (g)	32	22
Saturated Fat (g)	7	5
Sodium (mg)	890	540
Carbohydrate (g)	54	56
Fiber (g)	3	6
Protein (g)	16	17

Top This!

The next time you sink your teeth into a slice or two of pizza, consider what's on top. The saturated fat, calories, and sodium can quickly add up when you lay it on thick.

HERE'S WHAT TOPPINGS DELIVER

PIZZA TOPPING	CALORIES	TOTAL FAT (G)	SATURATED FAT (G)	SODIUM (MG)
Onions, ¼ cup	11	0	0	0
Broccoli Florets, ¼ cup	5	0	0	5
Red Bell Peppers, ¼ cup	10	0	0	0
Black Olives, ¼ cup	39	4	0	293
Chicken Breast, 1½ oz	70	2	0	31
Ham, 1½ oz	76	4	1	638
Extra Cheese, 1½ oz	135	10	7	176
Pepperoni, 1½ oz	135	13	5	523
Sausage, 1½ oz	157	13	5	550

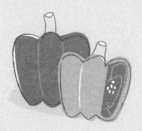

Squishy Squash Lasagna

MAKES 8 SERVINGS

Lasagna is like a sandwich; you can pretty much place any ingredient in between the layers and it works. A lot of lasagna recipes call for ground beef, sausage, and tons of cheese—making it hearty, but not so healthy. Janice and daughter Carolyn revamped this tried-and-true classic by incorporating butternut squash into the dish. Yes, you heard it here first folks: squash. And we're particularly proud of the results because the flavor, kid appeal, and good nutrition are through the roof.

Moms Make It Over By . . .

- Adding butternut squash for vitamins, minerals, phytonutrients, and fiber.
- Using part-skim cheeses and eliminating the high-fat meats to lower the saturated fat, sodium, and calories.

> One 20-ounce bag frozen butternut squash, thawed
>
> One 15-ounce carton part-skim ricotta cheese
>
> 2 large eggs
>
> ½ cup grated Parmesan cheese
>
> One 26-ounce jar pasta sauce
>
> One 9-ounce box oven-ready, no-boil lasagna noodles
>
> 2 cups preshredded part-skim mozzarella cheese

1. Place the squash in a food processor and pulse until completely pureed. Add the ricotta cheese, eggs, and Parmesan cheese and pulse a few turns until just combined.

2. Preheat the oven to 375°F.

3. To assemble the lasagna, spread ½ cup of pasta sauce on the bottom of a 9 x 13-inch baking pan. Place 4 noodles over the sauce, allowing them to overlap slightly. Leave about ¼-inch space between the noodles and the edges of the pan (because the lasagna will expand to the edges during cooking).

4. Continue layering by placing a third of the ricotta mixture (about 1½ cups), ½ cup mozzarella cheese, and ½ cup pasta sauce over the first noodle layer. Repeat the next two layers with the noodles, ricotta mixture, mozzarella cheese, and pasta sauce. End with 4 uncooked noodles, 1 cup pasta sauce, and ½ cup mozzarella cheese.

5. Cover with aluminum foil and bake until the mixture bubbles, 50 to 60 minutes. Let stand about 10 minutes before cutting. Top with extra Parmesan cheese if desired.

PREPARATION TIME: 15 MINUTES
COOKING TIME: 60 MINUTES

	Before	After
Calories	540	390
Fat (g)	34	14
Saturated Fat (g)	15	7
Sodium (mg)	1,140	650
Carbohydrate (g)	33	44
Fiber (g)	3	4
Protein (g)	26	25

Moms' Kitchen Notes: You can also make this recipe with one 10- or 12-ounce box of frozen pureed winter squash. Use your food processor or simply combine the ingredients in a large bowl with a spoon or electric beater.

Wagon Wheel Alfredo

MAKES 4 SERVINGS

A few years back, the Center for Science in the Public Interest (a nonprofit health-advocacy group in Washington, D.C.) declared fettuccine Alfredo a "heart attack on a plate." Their criticism may have been a bit harsh, but given the fact that Alfredo is often made with heavy cream, butter, and Parmesan cheese and has upwards of 50 grams of fat in a serving, we saw their point. To resuscitate this recipe, we skimmed away most of the artery-clogging saturated fat but kept the rich, time-honored flavors.

Moms Make It Over By . . .

🍓 Adding peas for vitamins, minerals, phytonutrients, and fiber.

🍓 Using lowfat milk and reduced-fat sour cream to lower the saturated fat and calories.

🍓 Using 2 ounces of dried pasta per serving to keep the portions and calories in check.

8 ounces dried small pasta wheels (about 3 cups)

1½ cups 1% lowfat milk

3 tablespoons all-purpose flour

⅔ cup grated Parmesan cheese

½ cup reduced-fat sour cream

4 ounces lean deli ham, diced

1½ cups frozen peas, thawed

Salt and pepper

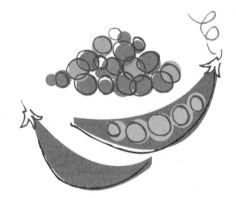

1. Cook the pasta according to package directions. Drain and set aside.

2. Return the saucepan to the stove (do not place over heat just yet). Add the milk and flour and whisk until well blended.

3. Place over medium-high heat and bring to a simmer, stirring constantly. Reduce the heat and continue to simmer and stir gently until the mixture thickens slightly, about 2 minutes.

4. Add the Parmesan cheese and sour cream and stir until well blended. Stir in the pasta, ham, and peas, and heat through. Season with salt and pepper to taste.

PREPARATION TIME: 10 MINUTES
COOKING TIME: 15 MINUTES

	Before	After
Calories	910	450
Fat (g)	54	11
Saturated Fat (g)	32	6
Sodium (mg)	990	630
Carbohydrate (g)	85	62
Fiber (g)	4	5
Protein (g)	25	27

Moms' Kitchen Notes: If you don't have lean deli ham on hand, use sliced, diced turkey instead.

Kitchen Sink Pasta Salad

MAKES 8 TO 10 SERVINGS

Whether you're heading to a backyard barbeque or need a cold dish for a hot summer's night, our Kitchen Sink Pasta Salad is an easy alternative to all those creamy macaroni salads sold at the supermarket deli counter. This salad is so versatile, you can add everything but the kitchen sink, and it's guaranteed to work every time.

Moms Make It Over By ...

- Adding broccoli and tomatoes for vitamins, minerals, phytonutrients, and fiber.
- Using lite salad dressing to lower the calories.
- Using about 2 ounces of dried pasta per serving to keep the portions and calories in check.

1 pound dried bow tie pasta

4 to 5 cups fresh or frozen broccoli florets

1 pint cherry or grape tomatoes (about 2 cups), sliced in half

One 14-ounce can artichoke hearts, drained, rinsed, and quartered, optional

6 to 8 ounces feta cheese, crumbled

3/4 cup pitted kalamata olives, chopped, or one 6-ounce can small black olives, drained

1/3 to 1/2 cup lite Italian or Caesar salad dressing

1/3 cup chopped fresh basil or cilantro, optional

1. Cook the pasta according to package directions. Five minutes before the pasta is done, add the broccoli. Bring back to a boil and cook until the pasta is done. Drain and place in a large bowl.

2. While the pasta is still warm, add the tomatoes, artichoke hearts as desired, cheese, olives, salad dressing, and herbs as desired and stir to combine.

3. Serve warm or refrigerate for a cold salad.

PREPARATION TIME: 15 TO 20 MINUTES

Moms' Kitchen Notes: You can also add bell pepper strips, canned chickpeas, or snow peas.

	Before	After
Calories	440	280
Fat (g)	26	9
Saturated Fat (g)	4	3.5
Sodium (mg)	800	500
Carbohydrate (g)	45	40
Fiber (g)	3	3
Protein (g)	6	10

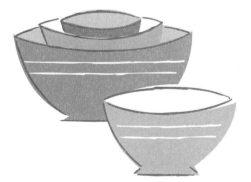

Eggplant Parm in a Pot

MAKES 4 TO 6 SERVINGS

Making eggplant Parmesan is time consuming and after all the effort, most kids don't even like it anyway. Maybe it's a texture thing. We devised an easier way to get eggplant Parmesan on the table in minutes. And since the eggplant is cut up into tiny pieces and then camouflaged in the pasta, it's a big hit with our kids.

Moms Make It Over By . . .

- Cooking in a moderate amount of healthy olive oil and using part-skim cheese to lower the saturated fat and calories.
- Using about 2 ounces of dried pasta per serving to keep the portions and calories in check.

> 8 ounces dried radiatore or other squiggly-shaped pasta (about 2 cups)
>
> 2 tablespoons olive oil
>
> 1 medium eggplant, peeled and cut into ¼-inch cubes (about 1 pound)
>
> 1 teaspoon dried basil
>
> 1 teaspoon garlic powder
>
> ½ teaspoon onion powder
>
> 2 cups pasta sauce
>
> 1 cup preshredded part-skim mozzarella cheese
>
> ⅓ cup grated Parmesan cheese
>
> 2 ounces sliced pepperoni, chopped, optional

1. Cook the pasta according to package directions. Drain, return to the pan, and set aside.

2. While the pasta is cooking, heat the oil in a large nonstick skillet over medium-high heat. Add the eggplant, basil, garlic powder, and onion powder, and cook, stirring frequently, until the eggplant becomes very tender, 8 to 10 minutes. Reduce the heat if the eggplant starts to stick to the skillet.

3. Add the cooked eggplant, pasta sauce, mozzarella cheese, Parmesan cheese, and pepperoni as desired to the pasta and stir to combine. Place over medium heat and stir until the pasta is heated through and the cheese melts, about 3 minutes.

PREPARATION TIME: 15 MINUTES
COOKING TIME: 15 MINUTES

	Before	After
Calories	640	360
Fat (g)	46	13
Saturated Fat (g)	14	4.5
Sodium (mg)	1,130	530
Carbohydrate (g)	36	45
Fiber (g)	7	5
Protein (g)	24	16

Moms' Kitchen Notes: Sauté sliced mushrooms with the eggplant if your family likes them.

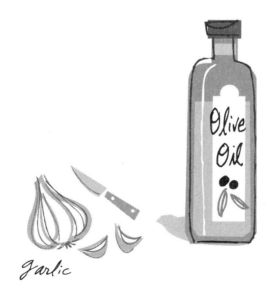

garlic

Thai Chicken Pizza

MAKES 4 TO 5 SERVINGS

As a young girl growing up in New York, Liz remembers riding her bike to the local pizzeria and ordering a slice of cheese pizza for 25 cents. Back then, pizza toppings were pretty basic. So basic, in fact, that Liz never imagined that 30 years later, she'd be creating a recipe for Thai Chicken Pizza. This deliciously easy pizza is a healthy alternative to some of the popular meat lover's pizzas now available at many national pizza chains.

Moms Make It Over By . . .

- Adding bell peppers for vitamins, minerals, phytonutrients, and fiber.
- Using part-skim cheese to lower the saturated fat and calories.

> 1 tablespoon peanut oil
>
> 8 ounces skinless, boneless chicken breast, cut into bite-size pieces
>
> 1 medium red bell pepper, cut into thin strips (about 1 cup)
>
> 1 medium yellow bell pepper, cut into thin strips (about 1 cup)
>
> ¼ cup Thai peanut sauce or peanut satay stir-fry sauce
>
> 1 tablespoon rice vinegar or white wine vinegar
>
> 1 large, partially baked, thin pizza crust
>
> 1 cup preshredded part-skim mozzarella cheese

1. Preheat the oven to 400°F.
2. Place a large baking sheet or pizza stone in the oven to preheat.
3. Meanwhile, heat the oil in a large nonstick skillet over medium-high heat. Add the chicken and cook 3 minutes. Add the bell peppers and cook until tender, about 5 minutes.
4. Stir in the peanut sauce and vinegar until well blended.

5. Spread the chicken mixture evenly over the pizza crust, top with the cheese, and carefully place on the baking sheet or pizza stone. Bake according to package directions, 8 to 10 minutes.

6. Slice and serve hot.

PREPARATION TIME: 15 MINUTES
COOKING TIME: 20 MINUTES

	Before	After
Calories	370	370
Fat (g)	22	13
Saturated Fat (g)	8	4.5
Sodium (mg)	860	510
Carbohydrate (g)	29	35
Fiber (g)	2	2
Protein (g)	15	27

Moms' Kitchen Notes: To shorten the prep time, use 2 to 3 cups frozen bell pepper strips instead of fresh ones.

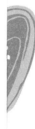

Cheeseburger Pizza

MAKES 6 SERVINGS

If your family loves meat and potatoes, chances are some of their favorite pizza toppings follow suit. Pizzas adorned with pepperoni, ground beef, sausage, and other such savory toppings are tough to resist, but they come with a price: more saturated fat and sodium than your cardiologist would ever recommend. The next time your family asks "Where's the beef?" serve it on these fun and nourishing little pizzas.

Moms Make It Over By . . .

- Adding bell pepper for vitamins, minerals, phytonutrients, and fiber.
- Switching to lean ground beef and part-skim cheese to lower the saturated fat and calories.
- Using whole grain English muffins for added nutrients and fiber.

> **One 12-ounce package whole wheat or oat bran English muffins (6 muffins)**
>
> **12 ounces lean ground beef (90% or higher)**
>
> **1 large red or orange bell pepper, finely chopped (about 1½ cups)**
>
> **½ teaspoon dried oregano or Italian seasoning**
>
> **1 cup pasta sauce**
>
> **1½ cups preshredded part-skim mozzarella cheese**

1. Preheat the oven to 400°F.

2. Slice the English muffins in half and place on a baking sheet. Toast lightly in the oven if desired. Set aside.

3. Place the beef, bell pepper, and oregano in a large nonstick skillet over medium-high heat and cook, breaking up the large pieces, until the meat is no longer pink, 6 to 8 minutes. Drain excess fat. Add the pasta sauce and mix well.

4. To assemble the pizzas, top each muffin half with a twelfth of the meat mixture. Sprinkle the cheese evenly over the top of each.

5. Bake until the cheese melts, 5 to 7 minutes. Serve hot.

PREPARATION TIME: 15 MINUTES
COOKING TIME: 15 MINUTES

Moms' Kitchen Notes: Use 1 pound ground meat if you like your pizzas a bit more meaty. Serve with a salad on the side.

	Before	After
Calories	550	300
Fat (g)	26	9
Saturated Fat (g)	12	4.5
Sodium (mg)	1,275	730
Carbohydrate (g)	55	32
Fiber (g)	3	6
Protein (g)	25	25

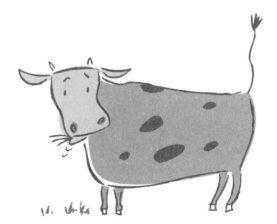

Pizza Bonita

MAKES 4 SERVINGS

If you love Mexican food, then you'll want to try our Pizza Bonita. It takes the best of Mexican food — refried beans, corn, and salsa — and brings them together in one amazing pizza. Since this simple recipe is 100 percent vegetarian, we decided to compare it to a few of the so-called healthy vegetarian pizzas now offered at some popular pizza chains. After crunching the numbers, we are happy to report that ours has a fraction of the saturated fat and mucho fewer calories.

Moms Make It Over By ...

🍓 Adding corn and salsa for vitamins, minerals, phytonutrients, and fiber.

🍓 Including refried beans for added nutrients and fiber.

🍓 Using reduced-fat cheese to lower the saturated fat and calories.

> One half of a 16-ounce can fat-free refried beans
>
> 1 large, partially baked, thin pizza crust
>
> ½ cup salsa
>
> 1½ cups frozen corn kernels, thawed
>
> 1 cup preshredded reduced-fat Mexican blend or Cheddar cheese
>
> One 2¼-ounce can sliced black olives, drained, optional

1. Preheat the oven to 450°F.

2. Place a large baking sheet or pizza stone in the oven to preheat.

3. Spread the refried beans evenly over the pizza crust and top evenly with the salsa, corn, cheese, and olives as desired. Place carefully on the baking sheet or pizza stone and bake according to package directions, 8 to 10 minutes.

4. Slice and serve hot.

PREPARATION TIME: 5 MINUTES
COOKING TIME: 10 MINUTES

	Before	After
Calories	610	380
Fat (g)	24	7
Saturated Fat (g)	10	2
Sodium (mg)	1,280	860
Carbohydrate (g)	75	59
Fiber (g)	6	6
Protein (g)	25	20

CHAPTER 9

Very Vegetarian

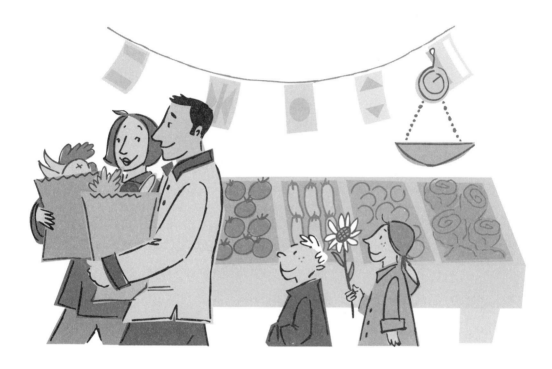

One-Pot Rice & Beans • Quick Quesadilla Pockets • No-Crabs-Allowed Cakes • Easy Enchilada Casserole • Mixed-Up Tofu • Tasty Tofu Nuggets • Peanut Butter (No Jelly) Noodles • Sunflower Zucchini Pie • Walnut Pasta Pancake • Shells with Soupy Lentil Sauce • Greek Goddess Mac & Cheese • Pups & Beans

They're everywhere. They live in our neighborhoods, hang out at our schools, and fill up at our corner gas stations. Some of them, including Chelsea Clinton, Martina Navratilova, and Paul McCartney, are also pretty famous. They're hard to spot because contrary to what some folks may think, vegetarians don't sit around eating bean sprouts all day nor do they wear Birkenstocks to black-tie affairs. The bottom line: Vegetarians don't look any different than the carnivores among us.

It turns out, however, that people who eat a well-planned vegetarian diet are different from non-vegetarians when it comes to their overall health. Research shows that vegetarians, in general, have a lower incidence of high blood pressure, high cholesterol levels, type 2 diabetes, and colon and lung cancers. They also live longer.

A vegetarian diet typically includes an abundance of fruits, vegetables, whole grains, beans, nuts, and lowfat dairy. But sometimes it can be lacking in variety and loaded with saturated fat. Take a teenager, for example, who comes home and announces to her mom that she's become a vegetarian. While giving up meat, fish, and poultry may seem like a good idea, if all she eats are potato chips, pizza, and pasta for dinner every night, she'll be missing out on a host of important nutrients.

The trick to planning a winning vegetarian diet is not intricate menu planning, nor is it restriction. It's variety. For years, experts believed it was crucial to eat combinations of protein foods, such as rice and beans, at the same meal in order to get all the essential amino acids into the diet (amino acids are the building blocks of protein). Today, we know that eating a mixture of protein foods throughout the day, versus at a single meal, will provide the complete protein you need.

Our goal with this chapter is to whet your appetite with updated versions of old vegetarian classics and to offer some new ideas for tasty meatless meals. We accomplished this with recipes like Sunflower Zucchini Pie (page 210). Instead of traditional quiche, made with a pie crust laden with 100-plus grams of fat, we created a delicious alternative with eggs (choose the omega-3 kind if you can find them), brown rice, zucchini, mozzarella cheese, and sunflower seeds. It's comfort food at its best. We also made tofu more appealing, giving you new ammunition to market this health-enhancing food to your family. We are confident that our Tasty Tofu Nuggets (page 206) and our Mixed-Up Tofu (page 204) will meet your demands for great flavor.

There's no rule that states you have to have meat at every meal. Going vegetarian a few nights a week can add variety to your dinner table and help you on your way to your meal makeover.

One-Pot Rice & Beans

MAKES 6 SERVINGS

What could be wrong with rice and beans? Well, not much. But as you've probably guessed by now, we are certified "overachievers" who never miss an opportunity to tinker with a recipe. The dish that we started with—made with rice, beans, and smoked sausage—was clearly a no-no for this chapter and the fact that it called for dried beans versus canned meant some serious streamlining was required.

Moms Make It Over By . . .

- Adding mixed vegetables for vitamins, minerals, phytonutrients, and fiber.
- Including reduced-fat cheese for bone-building calcium.

> 1¾ cups instant brown rice (about 3½ cups cooked)
>
> One 15½-ounce can black beans or kidney beans, drained and rinsed
>
> 2½ cups frozen mixed vegetables, thawed
>
> 1½ cups salsa
>
> 1½ cups preshredded reduced-fat Cheddar cheese
>
> ½ cup reduced-fat sour cream

1. Place the rice, 2 cups water, beans, vegetables, and salsa in a large saucepan or Dutch oven over high heat and stir until combined. Bring to a boil, reduce the heat, and simmer, covered, until most of the liquid is absorbed, 10 to 12 minutes.

2. Stir in the cheese until melted. Place in individual bowls and top with sour cream.

PREPARATION TIME: 5 MINUTES
COOKING TIME: 15 MINUTES

	Before	After
Calories	540	330
Fat (g)	17	5
Saturated Fat (g)	6	2.5
Sodium (mg)	1,030	630
Carbohydrate (g)	63	58
Fiber (g)	10	10
Protein (g)	31	18

Moms' Kitchen Notes: Serve with a crisp green salad.

Quick Quesadilla Pockets

MAKES 6 SERVINGS

Growing up, if our moms had given us quesadillas or enchiladas for dinner we would have said, "Huh?" Mexican food was a foreign cuisine back then but thankfully, it's mainstream today. However, with any cuisine, there's often a catch. Mexican food, with its beans, rice, and sizzling hot peppers, can be a health nut's delight. But pile on the cheese or get the deep-fat fryer going, as is often the case at fast food restaurants, and the amount of saturated and trans fats can quickly add up. Our homemade quesadillas put fast food to shame.

Moms Make It Over By . . .

- Adding bell pepper for vitamins, minerals, phytonutrients, and fiber.
- Using reduced-fat cheese and baking versus frying to lower the saturated fat, trans fats, and calories.
- Including beans for added nutrients and fiber.

> 1 tablespoon canola oil
>
> 1 large red bell pepper, finely diced (about 1½ cups)
>
> ½ teaspoon chili powder
>
> ½ teaspoon onion powder
>
> 1½ cups frozen corn kernels, thawed
>
> One 15½-ounce can pinto beans, drained and rinsed
>
> ½ cup salsa
>
> 2 cups preshredded reduced-fat Mexican blend or Cheddar cheese
>
> Six to eight 8-inch flour tortillas
>
> One 2¼-ounce can sliced black olives, drained, optional
>
> ½ cup reduced-fat sour cream, optional

1. Lightly oil or coat a large baking sheet with nonstick cooking spray and set aside.

2. Heat the oil in a large nonstick skillet over medium-high heat. Add the bell pepper, chili powder, and onion powder and cook until tender, about 5 minutes.

3. Preheat the oven to 400°F.

4. Add the corn, beans, salsa, and 1½ cups of the cheese to the skillet and cook until the mixture is heated through and the cheese melts, about 2 minutes.

5. To assemble the quesadillas, arrange the bean mixture evenly over half of each tortilla. Fold over, press down gently, and place each on the prepared baking sheet. Sprinkle the remaining cheese and olives as desired over the tortillas.

6. Bake until the cheese melts and the tortillas become crisp on the outside, about 10 minutes. Cut into quarters and serve. Top with sour cream as desired.

PREPARATION TIME: 10 MINUTES
COOKING TIME: 20 MINUTES

	Before	After
Calories	540	350
Fat (g)	30	9
Saturated Fat (g)	13	2
Sodium (mg)	1,150	630
Carbohydrate (g)	39	49
Fiber (g)	3	9
Protein (g)	19	18

Moms' Kitchen Notes: Any leftover vegetables from the night before can be chopped up and added to the quesadillas. Serve with extra salsa on the side for dipping.

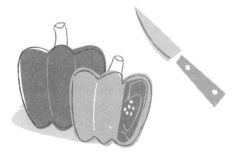

No-Crabs-Allowed Cakes

MAKES 4 SERVINGS (2 CAKES EACH)

Both of us have a rule at the dinner table: "No Crabs Allowed!" So when we decided to make a vegetarian version of crab cakes, our children came up with the funny name, No-Crabs-Allowed Cakes. Instead of using crab meat, gobs of mayonnaise, and butter for frying, we invented something a bit more healthful. These cakes are so good that whenever we make them, it puts everyone in a good mood.

Moms Make It Over By . . .

- Adding corn for vitamins, minerals, phytonutrients, and fiber.
- Using beans for added nutrients and fiber.
- Using light canola mayonnaise and cooking in a moderate amount of healthy olive oil to lower the saturated fat and calories.

> One 15½-ounce can cannellini beans, drained and rinsed
>
> 1 cup frozen corn kernels, thawed
>
> ¾ cup preshredded part-skim mozzarella cheese
>
> ¾ cup dried bread crumbs, divided
>
> 1 large egg, beaten
>
> ¼ cup light canola mayonnaise
>
> 1 tablespoon bottled or fresh lemon juice
>
> 1 teaspoon dried Italian seasoning
>
> ¼ teaspoon salt
>
> Pepper
>
> 1 tablespoon olive oil
>
> ½ to 1 cup pasta sauce, warmed

1. Mash the beans in a large bowl using the back of a large fork or spoon until smooth but still a bit chunky.

2. Add the corn, cheese, ½ cup of the bread crumbs, egg, mayonnaise, lemon juice, Italian seasoning, salt, and pepper to taste and mix well to combine.

3. Shape the mixture into eight ½-inch-thick patties and coat with the remaining bread crumbs.

4. Heat the oil in a large nonstick skillet over medium-high heat. Cook the patties until golden brown, about 4 minutes per side.

5. Serve with warm pasta sauce for dipping.

PREPARATION TIME: 15 MINUTES
COOKING TIME: 10 MINUTES

	Before	After
Calories	550	350
Fat (g)	33	13
Saturated Fat (g)	13	3
Sodium (mg)	1,270	710
Carbohydrate (g)	31	41
Fiber (g)	2	6
Protein (g)	31	16

Moms' Kitchen Notes: Serve with Sweet Potato Fries (page 304).

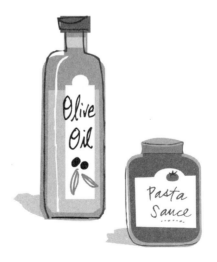

Easy Enchilada Casserole

MAKES 8 SERVINGS

Since this is a chapter devoted to vegetarian recipes, we figured the least we could do was add some vegetables. But a lot of the enchilada recipes out there don't include any. The recipe that we started with came from the back of a can of enchilada sauce. The list of ingredients was pretty meager: ground meat, enchilada sauce, cheese, and tortillas. The recipe was fatty and salty and a lot of fun to make over.

Moms Make It Over By . . .

- Adding bell peppers for vitamins, minerals, phytonutrients, and fiber.
- Using reduced-fat cheese and meat-free crumbles to lower the saturated fat and calories.
- Including beans for added nutrients and fiber.

> One 28-ounce can crushed tomatoes
>
> 1 tablespoon canola oil
>
> One 16-ounce bag frozen mixed bell pepper strips, thawed
>
> 2 teaspoons ground cumin
>
> 1 teaspoon chili powder
>
> 1 teaspoon onion powder
>
> 1 teaspoon garlic powder
>
> 1 teaspoon dried oregano
>
> ¼ teaspoon salt
>
> One 12- or 16-ounce bag meat-free or soy crumbles
>
> One 15½-ounce can black beans, drained and rinsed
>
> Twelve 6-inch corn tortillas
>
> 2 cups preshredded reduced-fat Cheddar cheese
>
> One 2¼-ounce can sliced olives, drained, optional
>
> ½ cup reduced-fat sour cream

1. Lightly oil or coat a 9 x 13-inch baking pan with nonstick cooking spray. Spread ¼ cup of the crushed tomatoes evenly over the bottom of the pan and set aside.

2. Heat the oil in a large nonstick skillet over medium-high heat. Add the bell peppers, cumin, chili powder, onion powder, garlic powder, oregano, and salt and cook until the peppers are tender, about 5 minutes.

3. Add the remaining crushed tomatoes, the meat-free crumbles, and beans and stir to combine. Cook, stirring frequently, for 5 minutes.

4. Preheat the oven to 400°F.

5. Arrange 6 tortillas on the bottom of the baking pan, allowing them to overlap. Top evenly with half the bean mixture and 1 cup of cheese. Arrange the remaining tortillas over the cheese. Top with the remaining bean mixture, cheese, and olives if desired.

6. Bake uncovered until the cheese melts and the casserole is heated through, about 20 minutes. Serve with sour cream.

PREPARATION TIME: 30 MINUTES
COOKING TIME: 20 MINUTES

	Before	After
Calories	570	320
Fat (g)	30	8
Saturated Fat (g)	13	3
Sodium (mg)	1,170	560
Carbohydrate (g)	47	43
Fiber (g)	2	10
Protein (g)	27	23

Moms' Kitchen Notes: If your family likes spicy food, add extra cumin and chili powder. Serve with sliced avocado on the side.

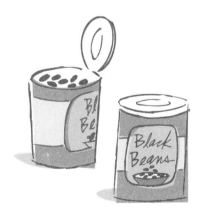

Mixed-Up Tofu

MAKES 4 SERVINGS

Liz's seven-year-old, Josh, is every dietitian's dream. He loves most foods . . . including tofu. It's not as though he packs it in his lunch box every day, but he's always happy when Mom makes it for dinner. The inspiration for this recipe came from a pork stir-fry in one of Liz's Asian cookbooks. She loved the taste but was a bit disappointed by the lack of vegetables. The recipe was easy to fix and with the addition of baby corn, even Liz's four-year-old, Simon, eats it.

Moms Make It Over By . . .

- Adding broccoli and corn for vitamins, minerals, phytonutrients, and fiber.
- Using tofu for less saturated fat and added nutrients such as heart-healthy soy protein.

6 ounces dried vermicelli pasta

One 14- or 16-ounce package extra-firm tofu, drained

2 tablespoons hoisin sauce

2 tablespoons lite soy sauce

1 tablespoon cornstarch

1 tablespoon peanut oil

One 16-ounce bag frozen broccoli florets, thawed, or 1 head broccoli, cut into small florets (5 to 6 cups)

One 15-ounce can small whole baby corn, drained and rinsed (cut in half if large)

1 teaspoon bottled crushed garlic, or 1 to 2 garlic cloves, minced

1 teaspoon ground ginger or 1 tablespoon bottled minced ginger

⅓ cup roasted cashews or peanuts, optional

1. Cook the pasta according to package directions. Drain and set aside.

2. Arrange several layers of paper towel on a cutting board. Place the tofu on the towels and cut into ½-inch cubes. Blot well with additional paper towels to absorb extra liquid.

3. Whisk together the hoisin sauce, soy sauce, and cornstarch in a bowl until well blended. Set aside.

4. Heat the oil in a wok or large nonstick skillet over high heat. Add the tofu, broccoli, corn, garlic, and ginger and stir-fry for 1 minute. Add ⅔ cup water, cover, and steam until the broccoli is tender, about 8 minutes. Stir occasionally.

5. Add the hoisin mixture to the wok (rewhisk if necessary), stir gently, and cook until the liquid thickens, about 2 minutes.

6. Serve in individual bowls over pasta and top with nuts as desired.

PREPARATION TIME: 15 MINUTES
COOKING TIME: 15 MINUTES

	Before	After
Calories	580	360
Fat (g)	25	10
Saturated Fat (g)	7	1.5
Sodium (mg)	680	580
Carbohydrate (g)	62	49
Fiber (g)	2	7 .
Protein (g)	25	21

Moms' Kitchen Notes: Many different vegetables work well in this dish. Try spinach, bok choy, asparagus, or carrots.

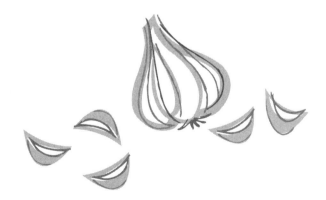

Tasty Tofu Nuggets

MAKES 3 SERVINGS

If your kids are keen on frozen chicken nuggets, but you're not keen on the greasy thick breading, try our vegetarian version made with tofu. Now, before you say, "No way, my kids would never eat that," consider that the main reason people don't "like" tofu is that they don't know how to cook it. Liz's neighbor, a converted Meal Makeover Mom, says this recipe is one of her vegetarian daughter's favorites.

Moms Make It Over By . . .

- Using tofu for added nutrients such as heart-healthy soy protein.
- Baking instead of frying.

> One 14- or 16-ounce package extra-firm tofu, drained
> 3 tablespoons lite teriyaki sauce
> 1 tablespoon lite soy sauce
> 1 tablespoon brown sugar
> 1 tablespoon sesame oil
> ½ teaspoon garlic powder
> ¼ teaspoon ground ginger
> ½ cup dried bread crumbs
> Sweet-and-sour sauce, optional

1. Arrange several layers of paper towel on a cutting board. Place the tofu on the towels and cut into bite-size cubes. Blot well with additional paper towels to absorb extra liquid.

2. Whisk together the teriyaki sauce, soy sauce, brown sugar, sesame oil, garlic powder, and ginger in a large, shallow bowl or dish. Add the tofu, toss to coat, and marinate for 5 minutes.

3. Preheat the oven to 425°F.

4. While the oven is heating, arrange the bread crumbs on a plate. Roll the tofu gently in the bread crumbs and coat evenly. Place the nuggets on a large baking sheet and cook until lightly browned, about 15 minutes. Serve with sweet-and-sour sauce if desired.

PREPARATION TIME: 15 MINUTES
COOKING TIME: 15 MINUTES

	Before	After
Calories	290	260
Fat (g)	21	11
Saturated Fat (g)	5	1.5
Sodium (mg)	470	500
Carbohydrate (g)	15	22
Fiber (g)	1	2
Protein (g)	10	17

Moms' Kitchen Notes: Serve with Orange Soup (page 112).

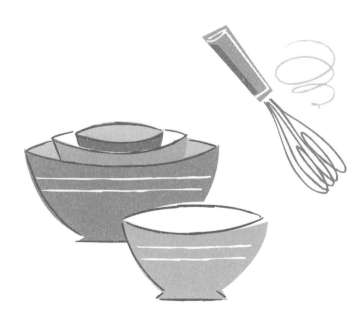

Peanut Butter (No Jelly) Noodles

MAKES 4 SERVINGS

Ask kids to list some of their favorite foods and most will say pasta and peanut butter. We offer the best of both worlds with this Asian-inspired peanut butter noodle dish. Instead of stopping at just the noodles, we added carrots and sweet bell peppers for good measure. Oh, and if you're wondering why the calories and fat are so obscenely high in the original recipe, it's from the 2 cups of peanut butter, 1 pound of pasta, and ½ cup of oil. Need we say more?

Moms Make It Over By . . .

- Adding carrots and bell pepper for vitamins, minerals, phytonutrients, and fiber.
- Using 2 ounces of dried pasta per serving to keep the portions and calories in check.
- Using a smaller portion of peanut butter and oil to lower the calories.
- Using lite soy sauce to lower the sodium.

    8 ounces dried bow tie pasta (about 3 cups)

    2 large carrots, cut in half lengthwise and sliced into ½-inch-thick half moons (about 2 cups)

    1 medium red bell pepper, sliced into very thin, 1-inch-long strips (about 1 cup)

    ⅓ cup creamy all-natural peanut butter

    ⅓ to ½ cup boiling water

    2 tablespoons lite soy sauce

    1 tablespoon toasted sesame oil

    1 tablespoon red wine vinegar

    ¾ teaspoon dried ginger

    ½ teaspoon garlic powder

    ¼ cup roasted peanuts, coarsely chopped

1. Bring a large saucepan of water to a boil. Add the pasta and carrots and cook according to package directions. Add the bell pepper 3 minutes before the pasta is done. Drain and return to the pan.

2. While the pasta is cooking, whisk together the peanut butter, boiling water, soy sauce, sesame oil, vinegar, ginger, and garlic powder in a medium bowl until well blended.

3. Add the peanut butter mixture to the pasta and stir to combine. Reheat if necessary.

4. Place in individual bowls and sprinkle with peanuts.

PREPARATION TIME: **15 MINUTES**
COOKING TIME: **15 MINUTES**

	Before	After
Calories	1,060	460
Fat (g)	69	20
Saturated Fat (g)	9	3.5
Sodium (mg)	1,260	430
Carbohydrate (g)	89	55
Fiber (g)	16	6
Protein (g)	29	16

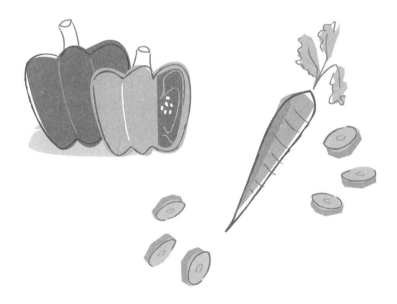

Sunflower Zucchini Pie

MAKES 5 SERVINGS

Quiche is one of those quintessential vegetarian dishes that everyone seems to love. But with all the shortening and butter in the crust and the heavy cream in the filling, a Meal Makeover Mom intervention was in order! Admittedly, our revamped recipe is a bit "out of the box" but, trust us, the combination of zucchini, cheese, brown rice, and crunchy sunflower seeds (an excellent source of heart-healthy vitamin E) makes a lot of sense once you try it.

Moms Make It Over By . . .

- Adding zucchini for vitamins, phytonutrients, and fiber.
- Using lowfat milk and reduced-fat cheese and making the quiche "crust-less" to lower the saturated fat and calories.
- Including brown rice and sunflower seeds for added nutrients and fiber.

1 tablespoon olive oil

1 medium zucchini, shredded (about 1½ cups)

1 teaspoon dried Italian seasoning

½ teaspoon bottled crushed garlic, or 1 garlic clove, minced

5 large eggs, beaten

1½ cups cooked instant brown rice

⅔ cup preshredded reduced-fat Cheddar cheese

½ cup 1% lowfat milk

⅔ cup Parmesan cheese, divided

¼ cup roasted, shelled sunflower seeds

½ teaspoon salt

1. Preheat the oven to 375°F.

2. Lightly oil or coat a 9-inch pie plate with nonstick cooking spray and set aside.

3. Heat the oil in a large nonstick skillet over medium-high heat. Add the zucchini, Italian seasoning, and garlic and cook until the zucchini is tender, about 5 minutes.

4. Place the eggs, rice, Cheddar cheese, milk, ⅓ cup Parmesan cheese, sunflower seeds, salt, and the cooked zucchini in a large bowl and stir to combine.

5. Pour the mixture into the prepared pie plate, top with the remaining ⅓ cup Parmesan cheese, and cook until golden brown, 30 to 35 minutes.

PREPARATION TIME: 15 MINUTES
COOKING TIME: 35 MINUTES

Moms' Kitchen Notes: Serve with a baby spinach salad.

	Before	After
Calories	610	300
Fat (g)	50	18
Saturated Fat (g)	28	6
Sodium (mg)	790	590
Carbohydrate (g)	32	18
Fiber (g)	1	2
Protein (g)	9	19

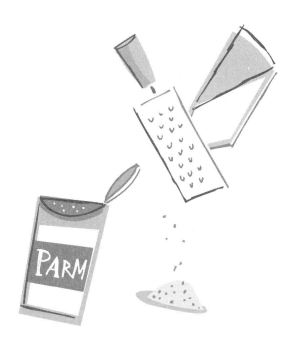

Walnut Pasta Pancake

MAKES 4 TO 5 SERVINGS

Whenever Liz has only 5 minutes to feed her family, she turns to her favorite standby: the simple cheese omelet. With a few extra minutes on her hands, however, she'll quickly whip up this super-nourishing giant pancake. We suggest you use omega-3 eggs in this dish so you and your family reap the additional health benefits.

Moms Make It Over By . . .

- Adding mixed vegetables for vitamins, minerals, phytonutrients, and fiber.
- Including walnuts for added nutrients and healthy omega-3 fats.
- Using whole wheat spaghetti for added nutrients and fiber.

3 ounces dried whole wheat spaghetti

6 large eggs, beaten

1½ cups frozen mixed vegetables, or frozen baby broccoli florets, thawed

½ cup grated Parmesan cheese

½ cup walnuts, toasted and coarsely chopped

½ teaspoon garlic powder

½ teaspoon onion powder

½ teaspoon salt

2 teaspoons canola oil

½ cup preshredded part-skim mozzarella cheese

1 cup pasta sauce, warmed

1. Cook the pasta according to package directions. Drain.

2. Combine the pasta, eggs, vegetables, Parmesan cheese, walnuts, garlic powder, onion powder, and salt in a large bowl and mix until well blended.

3. Heat the oil in a large nonstick skillet over medium heat. Add the egg mixture and flatten evenly with a spatula.

4. Cook until the bottom turns golden brown, 6 to 8 minutes. While the pancake is cooking, preheat the broiler.

5. Top the pancake evenly with the mozzarella cheese and place the skillet under the broiler. If the handle is plastic, wrap it in aluminum foil or slide the pancake carefully onto a large baking sheet. Broil until the top turns golden brown and the cheese melts, 3 to 4 minutes.

6. Slice and serve with warm pasta sauce for dipping.

PREPARATION TIME: 15 MINUTES
COOKING TIME: 15 MINUTES

	Before	After
Calories	340	410
Fat (g)	28	23
Saturated Fat (g)	14	6
Sodium (mg)	780	770
Carbohydrate (g)	1	29
Fiber (g)	0	7
Protein (g)	20	23

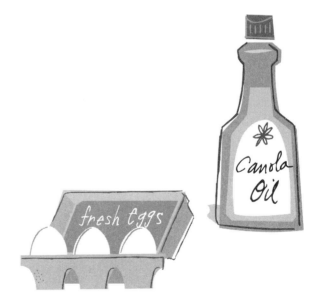

Shells with Soupy Lentil Sauce

MAKES 4 SERVINGS

If your hungry group of vegetarians is accustomed to eating plain old pasta with sauce night after night, shake things up a bit with our Shells with Soupy Lentil Sauce. Adding a can of lentil soup is easy, not to mention a novel way to get more iron, fiber, and protein-rich lentils into your family's diet.

Moms Make It Over By . . .

- Including a healthy lentil soup for added nutrients and fiber.
- Using 2 ounces of dried pasta per serving to keep the portions and calories in check.

> **8 ounces dried medium pasta shells (about 2½ cups)**
>
> **One 15-ounce can Health Valley Lentil & Carrot soup**
>
> **1 cup pasta sauce**
>
> **½ cup preshredded reduced-fat Cheddar cheese**
>
> **¼ cup grated Parmesan cheese**

1. Cook the pasta according to package directions. Drain and return to the pan.

2. Add the soup and pasta sauce to the pasta and simmer until heated through, about 3 minutes. Stir in the Cheddar cheese until melted.

3. Serve in individual bowls and top with Parmesan cheese.

PREPARATION TIME: 5 MINUTES

COOKING TIME: 15 MINUTES

	Before	After
Calories	480	310
Fat (g)	14	3.5
Saturated Fat (g)	5	1.5
Sodium (mg)	950	470
Carbohydrate (g)	64	56
Fiber (g)	9	7
Protein (g)	26	18

Pumping Iron

Many people believe that meat eaters are healthy and strong while vegetarians are all a bunch of weaklings walking around with iron-deficiency anemia. We're here to set the record straight. The most common nutritional problem among children is indeed iron-deficiency anemia, but the condition is just as likely to occur in kids who eat meat as in kids who don't.

Meat is rich in a type of iron called heme iron, while plant-based foods such as beans, tofu, iron-fortified breakfast cereals, and dried fruits contain nonheme iron. The difference between the two is the degree to which our bodies absorb them. It turns out that nonheme iron is not well absorbed . . . which may explain the concern over vegetarian diets. That said, however, research shows that eating foods rich in vitamin C along with iron-rich foods enhances absorption. So the bottom line for vegetarians: Plan well by drinking orange juice with your iron-fortified breakfast cereal, adding salsa to your Mexican bean burritos, and stir-frying broccoli with your tofu.

IRON-RICH PLANT-BASED FOODS

Black Beans

Chickpeas

Cream of Wheat

Instant Oatmeal

Lima Beans

Soymilk

Sunflower Seeds

Tofu

Wheat Germ

Whole Wheat Bread

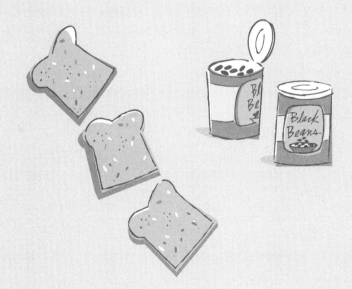

Greek Goddess Mac & Cheese

MAKES 6 SERVINGS

There are millions of mac & cheese recipes out there—not to mention the boxed stuff lining thousands of supermarket shelves—yet to our knowledge, no one has ever come up with a combo like this one! For this easy recipe, we combine sweet grape tomatoes, baby spinach, kalamata olives, and cheese, of course, for a Greek-style meal everyone loves.

Moms Make It Over By . . .

- Adding tomatoes and spinach for vitamins, minerals, phytonutrients, and fiber.
- Using lowfat milk and reduced-fat cheese to lower the saturated fat and calories.
- Using 2 ounces of dried pasta per serving to keep the portions and calories in check.

> 12 ounces dried spiral-shaped pasta such as gemelli or cavatappi (about 4 cups)
>
> 2¼ cups 1% lowfat milk
>
> 3 tablespoons all-purpose flour
>
> ¾ teaspoon garlic powder
>
> ½ teaspoon dried dill
>
> 2 cups preshredded reduced-fat Cheddar cheese
>
> ¼ cup grated Parmesan cheese
>
> One 6-ounce bag prewashed baby spinach (about 4 packed cups)
>
> One 1-pint container grape or cherry tomatoes, halved (about 2 cups)
>
> ½ cup kalamata olives, coarsely chopped, or one 2¼-ounce can sliced black olives, drained
>
> Salt and pepper
>
> ⅓ cup feta cheese, crumbled

1. Cook the pasta according to package directions.

2. While the pasta is cooking, whisk together the milk, flour, garlic powder, and dill in a medium saucepan until well blended. Place over medium-high heat and bring to a simmer, stirring constantly. Reduce the heat and continue to simmer and stir gently until the mixture thickens slightly, about 2 minutes.

3. Add the Cheddar cheese and Parmesan cheese and stir until the cheese melts. Remove from the heat and set aside.

4. When the pasta is done, drain and immediately return to the saucepan. Add the spinach and stir until wilted, 1 to 2 minutes. Add the tomatoes, olives, and cheese sauce and stir to combine. Reheat if necessary. Season with salt and pepper to taste.

5. Place in individual bowls and top with feta cheese.

PREPARATION TIME: 15 MINUTES
COOKING TIME: 15 MINUTES

Moms' Kitchen Notes: Serve with Chocolate-Dipped Strawberries for dessert (page 335).

	Before	After
Calories	510	440
Fat (g)	28	14
Saturated Fat (g)	17	7
Sodium (mg)	1,160	590
Carbohydrate (g)	42	53
Fiber (g)	2	3
Protein (g)	22	24

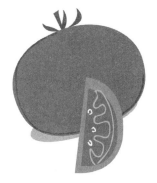

Pups & Beans

MAKES 6 SERVINGS

Janice has fond memories of her childhood birthdays, when Mom would let her choose the family meal for that night. Year after year, her request remained the same: hot dogs and beans. You see . . . even Janice has a dark side. Little did young Janice know that many hot dog products were loaded with salt, nitrites, and artificial colors and flavors. Today, as a dietitian, she often turns to the vegetarian-style dogs and still serves them with baked beans.

Moms Make It Over By . . .

- Switching to vegetarian hot dogs for added nutrients such as heart-healthy soy protein.
- Using vegetarian baked beans to lower the saturated fat.
- Including raisins for kid appeal and added nutrients and fiber.

One 28-ounce can vegetarian baked beans

6 tofu hot dogs, sliced into ¼-inch rounds

½ cup golden raisins

¼ cup ketchup

½ cup preshredded reduced-fat Cheddar cheese

1. Combine the beans, hot dogs, raisins, and ketchup in a medium saucepan and cook over medium-high heat, stirring frequently, until heated through, about 5 minutes.

2. Serve in individual bowls and top with cheese.

PREPARATION TIME: 5 MINUTES

COOKING TIME: 5 MINUTES

	Before	After
Calories	300	300
Fat (g)	16	4.5
Saturated Fat (g)	6	1.5
Sodium (mg)	1,190	540
Carbohydrate (g)	32	73
Fiber (g)	7	8
Protein (g)	12	19

Moms' Kitchen Notes: Serve with brown bread . . . a traditional New England favorite that comes in a can and is found near the baked beans.

CHAPTER 10

Here's the Beef & the Pork

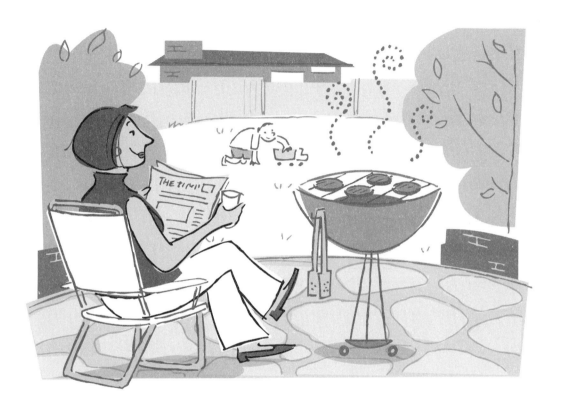

Cheesy Black Bean Burgers • Hunan Beef & Broccoli • Fiery Steak Fajitas • Mexican Lasagna • Creamy Stroganoff with Peas • Mini Meatballs with Whole Wheat Spaghetti • Have-It-Your-Way Tacos • Beef & Sweet Potato Stew • Hungry Kids Goulash • Snappy Pork Stir-Fry • Apricot-Glazed Grilled Pork • Granny Smith Pork Chops

Ground beef contributes more fat to the American diet than any other single food. It's no wonder there's been a nationwide stampede away from red meat. But believe it or not, beef contains a powerful bundle of nutrients that can promote good health. For starters, beef is rich in protein as well as iron, a mineral needed for strong blood and normal brain development. It's also an excellent source of the mineral zinc, important for a healthy immune system.

So given all the good news/bad news about beef, how can moms make it a more healthful addition to their family's diet? The answers are simple. First, stick to the USDA's recommended portion size of 3 to 4 ounces . . . that's the size of a cassette tape or a deck of cards. And second, choose the leanest cuts of red meat whenever possible. Look for tenderloin, sirloin, flank steak, and top round, and when you buy ground beef, go for 90%, 93%, or even 95% lean.

As for pork—which also gets a bad rap—producers have done an excellent job breeding skinnier pigs and hence slimmer cuts. The popular slogan touting pork as "the other white meat" makes a lot of sense given the fact that loin chops now have less fat than skinless chicken thighs and pork tenderloin is almost as lean as chicken breast meat.

For all of the beef and pork recipe makeovers presented in this chapter, we stick to the rules—smaller portions and leaner cuts. One of our favorites, Cheesy Black Bean Burgers (page 222), is a moist and delicious alternative to the basic cheeseburger. It has a scant 3 grams of saturated fat and an impressive 7 grams of fiber. The beans, by the way, are smashed up so your children may never even know they're in there. Another favorite is our Creamy Stroganoff with Peas (page 230). Besides slashing the saturated fat from 15 grams in a serving to a more respectable 7, we add peas for a kid-friendly vegetable in every bite.

Here's the beef & the pork, so eat up and enjoy.

The Leanest Ground Beef Money Can Buy

If you think 80% lean ground beef sounds like a health nut's dream come true, guess again. While 80% lean *implies* that 20% of the calories come from fat, you'll be surprised to learn that it really means 20% of the *weight* is fat. We think weights and percentages are confusing, so just look for the leanest ground beef money can buy. Your best bet is to stick with ground beef that is 90% lean or higher and to drain excess fat from your cooked ground beef.

BURGER BASICS

3-OUNCE COOKED HAMBURGER	CALORIES	SATURATED FAT (G)	TOTAL FAT (G)	% CALORIES FROM FAT
80% lean ground beef	216	5.3	13.7	57%
85% lean ground beef	204	4.8	12.2	54%
90% lean ground beef	182	3.8	9.4	46%
95% lean ground beef	148	2.4	5.4	33%

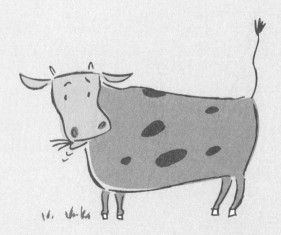

Cheesy Black Bean Burgers

MAKES 8 SERVINGS

When you're strapped for time and it's too hot to cook, burgers on the backyard grill are the perfect dinnertime solution. But when it comes to nutrition, hamburgers can be far from perfect, especially when they're made with fatty ground beef. Our easy makeover, with a fraction of the saturated fat and a lot more fiber, is truly a healthy indulgence.

Moms Make It Over By . . .

🍓 Switching to lean ground beef and reduced-fat cheese to lower the saturated fat and calories.

🍓 Replacing some of the meat with black beans for added nutrients and fiber.

One 15½-ounce can black beans, drained and rinsed

1 pound lean ground beef (90% or higher)

1 large egg, beaten

1 cup preshredded reduced-fat Cheddar cheese

⅓ cup seasoned bread crumbs

½ teaspoon garlic powder

8 hamburger buns

1. Preheat the grill to medium.

2. Place the black beans in a large bowl and mash with the back of a large spoon until smooth but still a bit chunky.

3. Add the beef, egg, cheese, bread crumbs, and garlic powder and mix until well combined.

4. Divide the beef mixture and shape into 8 patties.

5. Place the patties on the grill and cook until no longer pink inside and an instant-read thermometer registers at least 160°F, about 4 minutes per side.

6. Serve on hamburger buns with your favorite toppings and condiments.

PREPARATION TIME: 15 MINUTES
COOKING TIME: 10 MINUTES

Moms' Kitchen Notes: For burgers with an extra bite, add blue cheese or ½ teaspoon chili powder to the meat. You can also cook the burgers in a nonstick skillet over medium-high heat, about 4 minutes per side.

	Before	After
Calories	470	310
Fat (g)	28	8
Saturated Fat (g)	12	3
Sodium (mg)	610	510
Carbohydrates (g)	22	32
Fiber (g)	1	7
Protein (g)	32	28

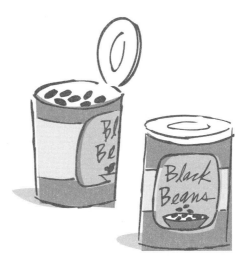

Hunan Beef & Broccoli

MAKES 4 TO 6 SERVINGS

Stir-fry dishes have the potential and reputation for being incredibly healthy, but the original recipe for this dish had so much soy sauce and oil that the sodium and fat levels were through the roof. We took care of those problems in no time flat and while we were at it added two powerhouse vegetables, broccoli and carrots. With them, you get a burst of beta-carotene, an antioxidant that may lower heart disease and cancer risk. Serve over Asian noodles or instant brown rice to complete the meal.

Moms Make It Over By . . .

- Adding carrots and broccoli for vitamins, minerals, phytonutrients, and fiber.
- Using lean flank steak to lower the saturated fat and calories.

    1 pound flank steak

    2 tablespoons lite soy sauce

    1 tablespoon rice vinegar or white wine vinegar

    1 tablespoon bottled minced ginger, or 1 teaspoon ground ginger

    1 tablespoon oyster sauce

    1 tablespoon toasted sesame oil

    1 tablespoon cornstarch

    1 teaspoon bottled crushed garlic, or 1 to 2 garlic cloves, minced

    1 tablespoon peanut oil or canola oil

    1 large head broccoli, cut into large florets, or one 16-ounce bag
        frozen broccoli florets, thawed

    2 to 3 large carrots, sliced very thin on the diagonal (2 to 3 cups)

    2 tablespoons hoisin sauce

1. Trim the meat of all visible fat. Cut the meat lengthwise with the grain into 3 equal strips, approximately 2 inches wide. Cut each strip across the grain into very thin slices. Set aside.

2. To make the marinade, place the soy sauce, vinegar, ginger, oyster sauce, sesame oil, cornstarch, and garlic in a medium bowl and mix well.

3. Add the meat and stir to coat. Set aside for 30 minutes or refrigerate for up to 24 hours.

4. Heat the peanut oil in a wok or large nonstick skillet over high heat. Add the meat and stir-fry until no longer pink, 5 to 8 minutes. Add 1 to 2 tablespoons of water if the meat sticks. Remove the meat to a plate and cover with foil to keep warm.

5. Add the broccoli, carrots, and ½ cup water to the wok, stir, and cover. Simmer until tender, 5 to 8 minutes.

6. Add the meat and hoisin sauce to the wok, stir to combine, and heat through, 1 to 2 minutes.

PREPARATION TIME: **25 MINUTES**
COOKING TIME: **20 MINUTES**

	Before	After
Calories	470	270
Fat (g)	39	13
Saturated Fat (g)	13	4
Sodium (mg)	850	630
Carbohydrate (g)	22	17
Fiber (g)	1	5
Protein (g)	22	22

Moms' Kitchen Notes: Chicken, pork, or tofu can be substituted for the beef. To speed up your dinner prep, slice and marinate the meat the night before.

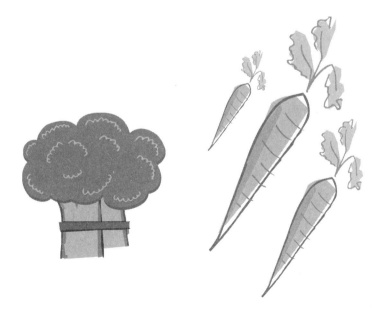

Fiery Steak Fajitas

MAKES 4 SERVINGS

If we told you that a fast food steak fajita has over 500 calories, 25 grams of fat, 1,200 milligrams of sodium, and little in the way of vegetables, you probably wouldn't lose sleep like we did. Okay, we're over it. And to prove it, we came up with our own homemade fajita recipe made with a virtual rainbow of colorful vegetables.

Moms Make It Over By...

- Adding bell peppers for vitamins, minerals, phytonutrients, and fiber.
- Using lean flank steak and reduced-fat sour cream to lower the saturated fat and calories.

> 2 teaspoons ground cumin
>
> 1 to 2 teaspoons chili powder
>
> 1 to 2 teaspoons curry powder
>
> ½ teaspoon garlic powder
>
> ¼ teaspoon salt
>
> 1 pound flank steak
>
> 1 tablespoon canola oil
>
> One 16-ounce package frozen bell pepper stir-fry mix, thawed
>
> Four 8-inch flour tortillas
>
> ½ cup salsa
>
> ¼ cup reduced-fat sour cream

1. Combine the cumin, chili powder, curry powder, garlic powder, and salt in a medium bowl. Set aside.

2. Trim the steak of all visible fat. Slice diagonally across the grain into very thin strips. Add to the spice mixture and stir until coated evenly.

3. Heat the oil in a large nonstick skillet over medium-high heat. Add the steak and the bell pepper mix and cook, stirring frequently, until the steak is no longer pink, about 7 minutes. Remove from the heat.

4. Stack the tortillas on a microwave-safe plate, uncovered, and heat in the microwave until warmed through, 30 to 45 seconds.

5. Divide the meat mixture evenly down the center of each tortilla and roll up. Serve with salsa and sour cream.

PREPARATION TIME: 10 MINUTES

COOKING TIME: 10 MINUTES

	Before	After
Calories	510	420
Fat (g)	25	17
Saturated Fat (g)	8	5
Sodium (mg)	1,200	590
Carbohydrate (g)	52	38
Fiber (g)	3	6
Protein (g)	21	27

Moms′ Kitchen Notes: Sliced avocado and chunks of ripe mango are ideal complements to the dish, adding extra vitamin C and fiber.

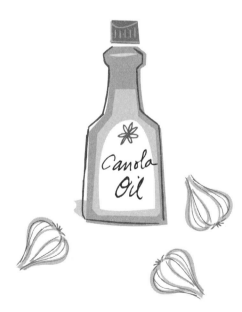

Mexican Lasagna

MAKES 8 SERVINGS

Who says lasagna has to be Italian? Our Mexican version, made with salsa instead of tomato sauce and tortillas instead of noodles, is always a big hit at dinnertime. The original recipe, given to Janice by her friend Mary, was bursting with flavor but had way too much sodium, thanks in part to the packet of salty taco seasoning mix.

Moms Make It Over By . . .

- Adding carrot and corn for vitamins, minerals, phytonutrients, and fiber.
- Switching to lean ground beef, reduced-fat cheese, and lowfat cottage cheese to lower the saturated fat and calories.
- Replacing the taco seasoning mix with a flavorful blend of spices and seasonings to lower the sodium.

> 1 pound lean ground beef (90% or higher)
> 1 large carrot, shredded (about 1 cup)
> One 16-ounce jar salsa
> One 15½-ounce can black beans, drained and rinsed
> One 10-ounce bag or box frozen corn kernels, thawed (about 2 cups)
> 1 teaspoon chili powder
> 1 teaspoon ground cumin
> Five 8-inch flour tortillas, cut in half
> One 16-ounce container lowfat cottage cheese
> 1½ cups preshredded reduced-fat Cheddar cheese

1. Cook the meat and carrot in a large nonstick skillet over medium-high heat, breaking up the large pieces, until no longer pink, about 5 minutes. Drain excess fat.

2. Preheat the oven to 375°F.

3. Add the salsa, black beans, corn, chili powder, and cumin to the skillet and stir to combine.

4. To assemble the lasagna, arrange a third (about 2 cups) of the meat mixture in a 9 x 13-inch baking pan. Layer half the tortillas over the meat, allowing them to overlap. Spoon half of the cottage cheese and ½ cup of the Cheddar cheese over the tortillas and spread evenly.

5. Place 2 more cups of meat mixture over the cottage cheese. Layer with the remaining tortillas and cottage cheese. End with the meat mixture.

6. Top with the remaining Cheddar cheese and bake uncovered until the cheese melts and the lasagna is heated through, about 25 minutes.

PREPARATION TIME: 20 MINUTES
COOKING TIME: 25 MINUTES

	Before	After
Calories	630	340
Fat (g)	29	7
Saturated Fat (g)	12	2.5
Sodium (mg)	1,820	880
Carbohydrate (g)	50	39
Fiber (g)	4	7
Protein (g)	40	30

Moms' Kitchen Notes: For a vegetarian option, use a bag of frozen non-meat or soy crumbles instead of beef.

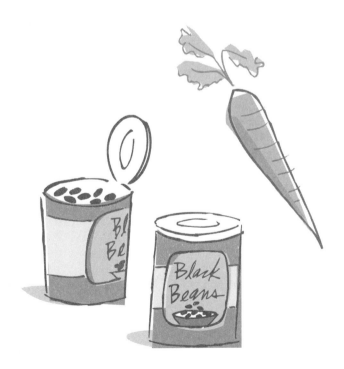

Creamy Stroganoff with Peas

MAKES 4 TO 5 SERVINGS

Classic beef stroganoff is one of those heavy-handed dishes made with butter and a lot of sour cream. Our lighter version is quick, easy, colorful, and exceptionally delicious. In fact, when we tested this recipe on a group of finicky ten-year-olds, they devoured every last bite. Shocking indeed!

Moms Make It Over By ...

- Adding peas for vitamins, minerals, phytonutrients, and fiber.
- Using lean sirloin steak and reduced-fat sour cream to lower the saturated fat and calories.
- Using about 2 ounces of dried pasta per serving to keep the portions and calories in check.

1 pound beef sirloin steak

6 to 8 ounces dried bow tie pasta (2¼ to 3 cups)

1 tablespoon olive oil

One 10-ounce package presliced mushrooms

1½ teaspoons onion powder

1 teaspoon garlic powder

¾ teaspoon salt

⅔ cup 1% lowfat milk

2 tablespoons all-purpose flour

1½ cups frozen peas, thawed

⅔ cup reduced-fat sour cream

¼ cup grated Parmesan cheese

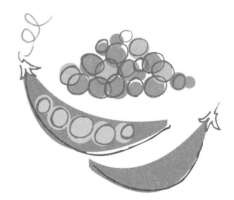

1. Trim the meat of all visible fat and cut diagonally across the grain into very thin strips. Set aside.

2. Cook the pasta according to package directions. Drain, return to the pan, and set aside.

3. While the pasta is cooking, heat the oil in a large nonstick skillet over medium-high heat. Add the steak, mushrooms, onion powder, garlic powder, and salt and cook, stirring frequently, until the steak is no longer pink and the mushrooms are tender, about 7 minutes.

4. Meanwhile, whisk together the milk and flour in a bowl until well blended.

5. Add the milk mixture and peas to the skillet and bring to a simmer, stirring frequently. Reduce the heat and continue to simmer and stir gently until the sauce thickens, 1 to 2 minutes.

6. Stir in the sour cream. Pour the mixture over the pasta and toss to combine. Serve in individual bowls and sprinkle with Parmesan cheese.

PREPARATION TIME: **15 MINUTES**
COOKING TIME: **15 MINUTES**

	Before	After
Calories	600	460
Fat (g)	32	18
Saturated Fat (g)	15	7
Sodium (mg)	830	610
Carbohydrate (g)	43	40
Fiber (g)	2	4
Protein (g)	35	33

Mini Meatballs with Whole Wheat Spaghetti

MAKES 6 SERVINGS

Since when have meatballs been considered healthy? Since we made them over. A lot of traditional meatball recipes are made with ground beef and ground pork and contain upwards of 30 grams of fat in a serving. Our meatballs are a lot leaner and just as appetizing.

Moms Make It Over By . . .

- Switching to lean ground beef to lower the saturated fat and calories.
- Using whole wheat spaghetti for added nutrients and fiber.
- Using about 2 ounces of dried pasta per serving to keep the portions and calories in check.

    1 pound lean ground beef (90% or higher)

    2 large eggs, beaten

    ¾ cup dried bread crumbs

    ¼ cup 1% lowfat milk

    ¼ cup grated Parmesan cheese

    1 tablespoon dried basil

    Pinch of pepper

    One 26-ounce jar pasta sauce

    10 to 12 ounces dried whole wheat spaghetti

1. Preheat the oven to 400°F.

2. Combine the meat, eggs, bread crumbs, milk, Parmesan cheese, basil, and pepper in a large bowl and mix well.

3. Shape the meat mixture into 35 to 40 small meatballs.

4. Place the meatballs on a baking sheet and cook until lightly browned, 10 minutes.

5. Meanwhile, place the pasta sauce in a large saucepan over medium heat, cover, and bring to a simmer. When the meatballs are done, add to the sauce, reduce the heat, and simmer, covered, about 20 minutes.

6. While the meatballs are simmering, cook the pasta according to package directions. Drain and transfer to a large serving bowl. Top with the meatballs and pasta sauce, mix together, and serve.

PREPARATION TIME: 15 MINUTES
COOKING TIME: 30 MINUTES

Moms' Kitchen Notes: Serve with Garlicky Sautéed Spinach (page 316).

	Before	After
Calories	610	390
Fat (g)	30	9
Saturated Fat (g)	11	3
Sodium (mg)	1,330	640
Carbohydrate (g)	55	54
Fiber (g)	5	8
Protein (g)	31	29

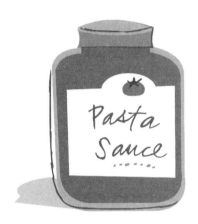

Have-It-Your-Way Tacos

MAKES 6 SERVINGS

A lot of supermarket products today are designed to make life easier in the kitchen. While we are all for convenience, some of those items come with a lot of "extra" ingredients that you may not want to serve your family. Take taco kits, for example. They often contain a dozen taco shells, a packet of taco seasoning mix, 1/2 cup of sauce, and ingredients like monosodium glutamate and hydrogenated vegetable oils. We say, why bother? Our naturally delicious and equally simple recipe uses common spices right from your own cupboard, your own choice of taco shells, and 1 cup of salsa, a good source of the anti-cancer antioxidant lycopene.

Moms Make It Over By . . .

- Switching to lean ground beef and reduced-fat cheese to lower the saturated fat.
- Replacing the taco seasoning mix with a flavorful blend of spices and seasonings to lower the sodium.
- Using taco shells made without hydrogenated vegetable oils to eliminate the trans fats.
- Including beans for added nutrients and fiber.

    1 pound lean ground beef or turkey (90% lean or higher)

    12 taco shells

    One 15½-ounce can black beans, drained and rinsed

    1½ cups preshredded reduced-fat Cheddar cheese

    1 cup salsa

    2 teaspoons ground cumin

    1 teaspoon chili powder

    ½ teaspoon garlic powder

PICK-AND-CHOOSE TOPPINGS (OPTIONAL)

1 avocado, peeled, pitted, and chopped

1 tomato, chopped

½ cup reduced-fat sour cream

1 cup shredded lettuce

½ cup sliced black olives

	Before	After
Calories	370	310
Fat (g)	21	11
Saturated Fat (g)	7	3
Sodium (mg)	800	630
Carbohydrate (g)	25	25
Fiber (g)	3	6
Protein (g)	21	27

1. Preheat the oven to 350°F.

2. Heat a large nonstick skillet over medium-high heat. Add the meat and cook, breaking up the large pieces, until no longer pink, about 5 minutes. Drain excess fat.

3. While the meat is cooking, bake the taco shells according to package directions.

4. When the meat is done, add the beans, cheese, salsa, cumin, chili powder, and garlic powder and stir to combine. Cook until heated through and the cheese melts, about 2 minutes.

5. Spoon 3 to 4 tablespoons of the meat filling into each of 12 taco shells. Serve with optional toppings.

PREPARATION TIME: 10 MINUTES
COOKING TIME: 10 MINUTES

Moms' Kitchen Notes: Leftover filling can be used the next day for a quick wrap.

Beef & Sweet Potato Stew

MAKES 6 SERVINGS

Bored with beef stew? Tired of the same old recipe with white potatoes and carrots? If you're looking for a new flavor experience, then you've got to try our Beef & Sweet Potato Stew. We like this recipe makeover for two reasons. First, the sweet potatoes and dried plums (aka prunes) in this dish are teeming with powerful disease-fighting antioxidants. And second, the stew is sweet and delicious and kids just love it.

Moms Make It Over By ...

- Adding mushrooms, sweet potatoes, green beans, and dried plums for vitamins, minerals, phytonutrients, and fiber.
- Using a smaller portion of meat and more vegetables to lower the saturated fat and calories.

> ¼ cup all-purpose flour
>
> 1¼ pounds lean stew meat, trimmed of visible fat and cut into ¾-inch cubes
>
> 2 tablespoons olive oil or canola oil
>
> 1 small onion, cut into 1-inch wedges
>
> One 10-ounce package presliced mushrooms
>
> 2 large sweet potatoes, peeled and cut into 1-inch cubes (about 6 cups)
>
> 2 cups all-natural beef broth or chicken broth
>
> One 8-ounce can tomato sauce
>
> 10 pitted dried plums, quartered
>
> ½ teaspoon salt
>
> ½ teaspoon garlic powder
>
> ¼ teaspoon ground cinnamon
>
> ⅛ teaspoon ground cloves
>
> 2 cups frozen cut green beans, thawed
>
> Salt and pepper

1. Place the flour in a bowl. Add the beef, toss until coated, and shake off excess.

2. Heat 1 tablespoon of the oil in a large saucepan or Dutch oven over medium-high heat. Add the beef cubes and cook, stirring occasionally, until lightly browned, 3 to 5 minutes. Remove to a bowl and set aside.

3. Add the remaining oil, onion, and mushrooms to the saucepan. Add a few tablespoons of water or broth and scrape up any brown bits that may have stuck to the bottom. Stir frequently and cook until the onions and mushrooms are tender, about 5 minutes.

4. Return the beef and any accumulated juices to the pan. Add the sweet potatoes, broth, tomato sauce, plums, salt, garlic powder, cinnamon, and cloves. Bring to a boil, reduce the heat, and simmer, covered, for 30 minutes.

5. Stir in the green beans and simmer, uncovered, until the sweet potatoes and green beans are tender, 20 to 30 additional minutes. Season with salt and pepper to taste.

PREPARATION TIME: **20 MINUTES**
COOKING TIME: **1 HOUR 10 MINUTES**

	Before	After
Calories	530	340
Fat (g)	21	12
Saturated Fat (g)	8	3
Sodium (mg)	660	660
Carbohydrate (g)	50	38
Fiber (g)	6	6
Protein (g)	31	23

Moms' Kitchen Notes: Serve with Honey Wheat Popovers (page 308).

Hungry Kids Goulash

MAKES 4 TO 6 SERVINGS

Our Hungry Kids Goulash is a takeoff on Hungarian Goulash . . . a slow-cooked stew traditionally made with beef and vegetables and then flavored with Hungarian paprika. But instead of spending hours waiting for your dinner to cook, our new-and-improved recipe is designed to get you in and out of the kitchen in a matter of minutes. For the vegetables, we chose carrots and corn. Oh, and by the way, if you think corn is just one of those starchy vegetables with little nutritional value, research now shows that corn contains two important antioxidants, lutein and zeaxanthin, shown to protect against eye diseases such as cataracts and macular degeneration.

Moms Make It Over By . . .

- Adding carrot and corn for vitamins, minerals, phytonutrients, and fiber.
- Switching to lean ground beef to lower the saturated fat and calories.
- Using about 2 ounces of dried pasta per serving to keep the portions and calories in check.

8 ounces dried egg noodles (about 4 cups)
1 pound lean ground beef (90% or higher)
1 large carrot, shredded (about 1 cup)
2 cups frozen corn kernels, thawed
One 26-ounce jar pasta sauce
¼ cup grated Parmesan cheese

1. Cook the pasta according to package directions. Drain and return to the pan.

2. While the pasta is cooking, place the meat and carrot in a large nonstick skillet over medium-high heat. Cook, breaking up the large pieces, until no longer pink, about 5 minutes. Drain excess fat.

3. Add the corn and pasta sauce and stir to combine. Cook until heated through, 2 to 3 minutes.

4. Stir the meat mixture into the pasta. Serve in individual bowls and sprinkle with Parmesan cheese.

PREPARATION TIME: 5 MINUTES
COOKING TIME: 10 MINUTES

Moms' Kitchen Notes: Serve with a crisp green salad.

	Before	After
Calories	530	370
Fat (g)	22	8
Saturated Fat (g)	8	3
Sodium (mg)	850	460
Carbohydrate (g)	52	48
Fiber (g)	4	5
Protein (g)	30	28

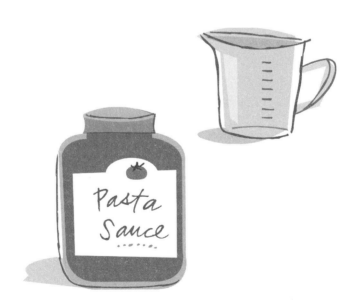

Snappy Pork Stir-Fry

MAKES 4 SERVINGS

Our inspiration for this recipe came from sweet and sour pork, but instead of a lot of pork, a thick gooey sauce, and only a few overcooked green bell peppers, we transformed it into a colorful and quick stir-fry. If your children have never tasted a snow pea before . . . now's their chance.

Moms Make It Over By . . .

- 🍓 Adding carrots and snow peas for vitamins, minerals, phytochemicals, and fiber.
- 🍓 Using a lean cut of pork to lower the saturated fat.

> 1 pound boneless center cut pork chops or pork tenderloin
>
> 1 cup orange juice
>
> ¼ cup packed brown sugar
>
> 2 tablespoons lite soy sauce
>
> 1 tablespoon cornstarch
>
> 1 tablespoon hoisin sauce
>
> ½ teaspoon ground ginger
>
> ½ teaspoon garlic powder
>
> 4 teaspoons toasted sesame oil
>
> 2 to 3 large carrots, sliced thin on the diagonal (2 to 3 cups)
>
> One 6-ounce box frozen snow peas, thawed
>
> ½ cup cashews

1. Trim the pork of all visible fat, slice into very thin strips, and set aside.

2. Whisk together the orange juice, brown sugar, soy sauce, cornstarch, hoisin sauce, ginger, and garlic powder in a medium bowl until well blended. Set aside.

3. Heat 2 teaspoons of the oil in a large nonstick skillet or wok over medium-high heat. Add the pork and cook, stirring frequently, until no longer pink, 3 to 5 minutes. Remove the pork to a plate and cover with foil to keep warm.

4. Add the remaining oil to the skillet. Add the carrots and stir-fry until crisp-tender, about 5 minutes. Add the snow peas and cook an additional 1 minute until heated through.

5. Rewhisk the orange juice mixture and add to the skillet with the cooked pork and cashews. Bring to a simmer, stirring constantly. Continue to simmer and stir gently until the mixture thickens slightly, about 2 minutes.

PREPARATION TIME: 15 MINUTES
COOKING TIME: 15 MINUTES

	Before	After
Calories	430	430
Fat (g)	22	18
Saturated Fat (g)	7	4
Sodium (mg)	510	490
Carbohydrate (g)	25	39
Fiber (g)	<1	4
Protein (g)	32	28

Moms' Kitchen Notes: Serve over instant brown rice or Asian noodles with Mandarin oranges on the side.

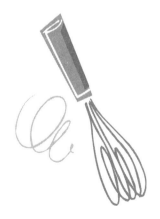

Apricot-Glazed Grilled Pork

MAKES 4 SERVINGS

For a healthier change of pace from pork roast and gravy, try our easy-to-make Apricot-Glazed Grilled Pork. Besides the fact that it's a lot leaner, it's also a lot faster. A typical pork roast takes an hour or more to cook, while our dish can be on the table in under 30 minutes.

Moms Make It Over By ...

🍓 Using pork tenderloin and nixing the gravy in favor of an apricot-mustard glaze to lower the saturated fat and calories.

> ¼ cup all-fruit apricot jam
>
> ¼ cup honey mustard
>
> 1 pound pork tenderloin
>
> ¼ teaspoon salt
>
> ⅛ teaspoon pepper

1. Preheat the grill to medium-high.

2. Combine the jam and mustard in a small bowl and set aside.

3. Trim the pork of all visible fat and season with salt and pepper.

4. Place the pork on the grill and cook for about 8 minutes. Turn the pork and brush the top with the apricot glaze. Cook another 6 to 8 minutes, turn again, and brush with the remaining glaze.

5. Continue cooking until the pork is still slightly pink in the center and an instant-read thermometer registers 160°F, an additional 2 to 3 minutes.

PREPARATION TIME: 10 MINUTES
COOKING TIME: 20 MINUTES

	Before	After
Calories	460	230
Fat (g)	31	7
Saturated Fat (g)	12	1.5
Sodium (mg)	650	210
Carbohydrate (g)	11	20
Fiber (g)	0	0
Protein (g)	34	23

Moms' Kitchen Notes: To cook in the oven, bake at 400°F until an instant-read thermometer registers 160°F, about 25 minutes.

Skinny Cuts of Meat

Beef and pork are considered taboo with many health-conscious families, yet the USDA classifies eight cuts of beef and eight cuts of pork as lean. The following chart compares the fat and saturated fat content of a 3-ounce cooked portion of various cuts of meat trimmed of visible fat. Notice how all of the cuts listed below have less total fat than skinless chicken thighs.

3-OUNCE PORTION	SATURATED FAT (G)	TOTAL FAT(G)
CHICKEN CUTS		
Skinless Chicken Breast	0.9 g	3.0 g
Skinless Chicken Thigh	2.6 g	9.2 g
PORK CUTS		
Pork Tenderloin	1.4 g	4.1 g
Boneless Loin Roast	2.2 g	6.1 g
Boneless Center Cut Chops	2.9 g	8.3 g
BEEF CUTS		
Eye of Round/Top Round	1.4 g	4.2 g
Top Sirloin	2.4 g	6.1 g
Bottom Round	2.1 g	6.3 g
Tenderloin	3.0 g	8.1 g
Flank Steak	3.7 g	8.6 g

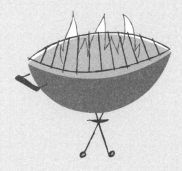

Granny Smith Pork Chops

MAKES 4 SERVINGS

Breaded pork chops fried in oil and then smothered in gravy is one of those hearty, old-fashioned meals that many moms—and their families—have always adored. But unfortunately, this dish is a far cry from heart-healthy. Our modern takeoff replaces the high-fat gravy with something a whole lot lighter and even more delicious.

Moms Make It Over By . . .

- Adding apple for vitamins, phytonutrients, and fiber.
- Using a lean cut of pork and creating a fruit-based topping to lower the saturated fat and calories.
- Including pecans for added nutrients and heart-healthy monounsaturated fats.

1 pound boneless, thin-sliced lean pork chops

1 tablespoon canola oil

1 large Granny Smith apple, cut into ½-inch cubes (about 2 cups)

1 cup apple juice

¼ cup golden raisins

2 tablespoons brown sugar

1 tablespoon bottled or fresh lemon juice

½ teaspoon salt

¼ teaspoon ground cinnamon

1 tablespoon cornstarch

2 tablespoons water or apple juice

¼ cup pecans, toasted and coarsely chopped

1. Trim the meat of all visible fat.

2. Heat the oil in a large nonstick skillet or Dutch oven over medium-high heat. Add the pork and cook until golden brown, 1 to 2 minutes per side.

3. Add the apple, apple juice, raisins, brown sugar, lemon juice, salt, and cinnamon and stir to combine. Bring to a boil, reduce the heat, and simmer, covered, until the apples are tender, 10 to 15 minutes.

4. Meanwhile, combine the cornstarch and water in a small bowl and stir until well blended. Add to the skillet and simmer, stirring constantly, until the mixture thickens, about 2 minutes.

5. Stir in the pecans and serve.

PREPARATION TIME: **15 MINUTES**
COOKING TIME: **20 MINUTES**

	Before	After
Calories	460	330
Fat (g)	33	14
Saturated Fat (g)	14	2.5
Sodium (mg)	1,070	340
Carbohydrate (g)	10	27
Fiber (g)	0	2
Protein (g)	28	23

Moms' Kitchen Notes: Serve with egg noodles and a colorful vegetable.

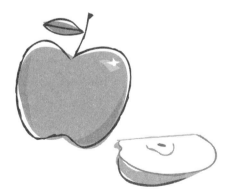

CHAPTER 11

Hooked on Seafood

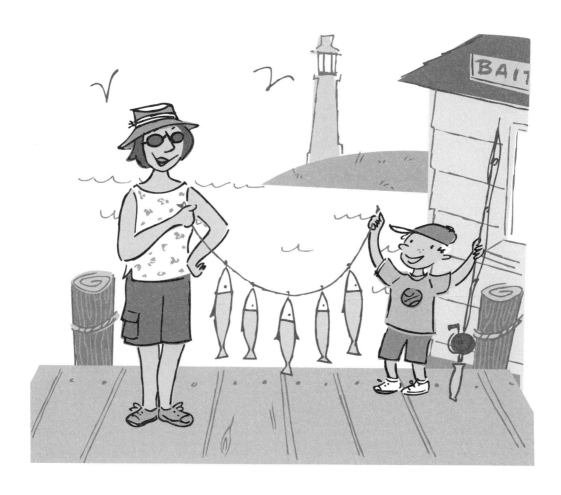

Flaky Fish Sticks • Tuna Twist Casserole • Corny Tuna Cakes • Linguine with Clam Sauce • Grilled Salmon with Ginger Honey Glaze • Walnut-Crusted Salmon • Shrimp Curry in a Hurry • Sweet & Slightly Sour Shrimp • Shrimp "Not-So-Fried" Rice • Almond Battered Fish • Baked Fish with Spinach Cheese Sauce • Cheesy Pecan Fish Rolls

Tilapia, perch, smelt, rockfish, and roughy are less popular than cod and salmon, but there's no denying the fact that fish, no matter the name, is amazingly good for our health. For starters, seafood is an excellent source of high-quality protein. It's also low in saturated fat, the type that can raise cholesterol levels. As an added benefit, some fish, namely salmon, mackerel, tuna, and other cold-water varieties, are rich in omega-3 fatty acids. Research shows that this important polyunsaturated fat may play a key role in reducing heart disease risk, lowering blood pressure, alleviating the symptoms of rheumatoid arthritis and depression, and promoting eye and brain development in babies. It's no wonder the American Heart Association recommends eating 2 servings of fish a week.

All the good news on seafood may be enough motivation for some adults to increase their intake, but it's often a tougher sell with kids. If you tell your children to eat more fish so they don't have a heart attack when they're sixty, they may look at you like you have three heads (one more than the two they already think you have). With the exception of canned tuna and fish sticks, children often turn their noses up when seafood is served.

Let's face it. If it's not cooked right, fish can be bland and boring, not to mention dry. Seafood can also be a saturated fat trap when it's smothered in a rich cream sauce and butter or breaded and deep-fat fried. Our challenge in this chapter, therefore, was to create twelve healthy and mouthwatering recipes to inspire home cooks to make fish a bigger part of their family's diet. You'll love our home-made version of store-bought fish sticks—Flaky Fish Sticks (page 248)—made with a crispy coating of corn flakes but none of the cholesterol-raising hydrogenated oils found in many commercial products. If sweet and sour shrimp happens to be one of your family's favorites, you'll be amazed when you try our simple makeover. Sweet & Slightly Sour Shrimp (page 262) has a fraction of the fat and sodium in the original recipe and instead of a paltry 1/4 cup diced green peppers, we add heaping cups of milder vegetables kids love.

For moms who think dishes like our Shrimp Curry in a Hurry (page 260) and Linguine with Clam Sauce (page 254) are for grown-ups only, we encourage you to try them. One bite and you and your family are sure to be hooked on more seafood.

Flaky Fish Sticks

MAKES 4 SERVINGS

You can't beat the convenience or the kid appeal of frozen fish sticks. In fact, we usually keep a box or two in the freezer for those hectic nights when we're too tired to cook. But if you hang out in supermarkets like we do and read the ingredients used in many of the commercial brands, you'll notice the words "partially hydrogenated vegetable oil" . . . a red flag that the product contains cholesterol-raising trans fatty acids. When time permits, try our easy Flaky Fish Sticks. Your kids may never go back to eating the frozen kind. Sorry!

Moms Make It Over By . . .

- Using less breading and more fish to increase the high-quality protein.
- Coating the fish in canola oil and a corn flake breading to eliminate the trans fats.

2 cups corn flakes

¼ cup grated Parmesan cheese

½ teaspoon garlic powder

¼ teaspoon salt

3 tablespoons canola oil

1¼ pounds firm white fish such as cod or halibut, cut into ½- to ¾-inch-thick "sticks"

1. Preheat the oven to 500°F.
2. Lightly oil or coat a large baking sheet with nonstick cooking spray and set aside.
3. Place the corn flakes in a resealable plastic bag and crush to a fine texture using a rolling pin or the bottom of a small saucepan, or place in a food processor and pulse several turns until finely crushed.
4. Combine the corn flakes, Parmesan cheese, garlic powder, and salt in a medium bowl and mix well.
5. Place the oil in a small bowl. Lightly coat each piece of fish in the oil, then coat evenly with the corn flake mixture.

6. Arrange the fish on the prepared baking sheet and bake until golden brown, about 10 minutes.

PREPARATION TIME: 20 MINUTES
COOKING TIME: 10 MINUTES

Moms' Kitchen Notes: Serve with Maple-Glazed Carrots (page 313).

	Before	After
Calories	290	270
Fat (g)	17	13
Saturated Fat (g)	2.5	2
Sodium (mg)	560	420
Carbohydrate (g)	23	12
Fiber (g)	0	0.5
Protein (g)	10	25

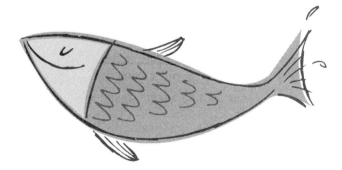

Tuna Twist Casserole

MAKES 6 TO 8 SERVINGS

Recipes for tuna noodle casserole appear in almost every family cookbook. Many call for heavy cream or canned cream of mushroom soup. Some recipes even include crushed potato chips . . . for the topping, of course. To revamp this 1940s classic, we added a new twist by using antioxidant-rich tomato soup and tossing in some colorful little green peas.

Moms Make It Over By . . .

- Adding peas for vitamins, minerals, phytonutrients, and fiber.
- Switching to reduced-sodium tomato soup to lower the saturated fat and sodium.
- Using about 2 ounces of dried pasta per serving to keep the portions and calories in check.

1½ cups corn flakes

12 ounces dried cavatappi or other twisty-shaped pasta (about 4 cups)

Two 10¾-ounce cans 30%-less-sodium tomato soup

Two 6-ounce cans solid white, water-packed tuna, drained and flaked

2 cups frozen peas, thawed

1½ cups preshredded part-skim mozzarella cheese

¼ cup grated Parmesan cheese

1. Lightly oil or coat a 9 x 13-inch baking pan with nonstick cooking spray and set aside.

2. Place the corn flakes in a resealable plastic bag and crush to a coarse texture using a rolling pin or the bottom of a small saucepan, or place in a food processor and pulse a few turns until coarsely crushed. Set aside.

3. Preheat the oven to 375°F.

4. Cook the pasta according to package directions, drain, and return to the pan. Stir in the soup, tuna, peas, and mozzarella cheese. Arrange in the baking pan.

5. Sprinkle the Parmesan cheese and corn flakes evenly over the top and bake uncovered until the mixture bubbles and the top turns golden brown, about 15 minutes.

PREPARATION TIME: 20 MINUTES
COOKING TIME: 15 MINUTES

Moms' Kitchen Notes: Serve with sliced oranges or melon.

	Before	After
Calories	410	410
Fat (g)	19	9
Saturated Fat (g)	8	4.5
Sodium (mg)	1,050	470
Carbohydrate (g)	34	53
Fiber (g)	2	4
Protein (g)	26	29

Mercury and Seafood

Certain fish may contain high levels of mercury. Therefore, according to the FDA, pregnant women and women of childbearing age should not eat large predator fish, including shark, swordfish, king mackerel, and tilefish. Mercury can be harmful to the developing nervous system of an unborn child. It is also prudent for nursing mothers and young children to avoid these fish.

Corny Tuna Cakes

MAKES 4 SERVINGS

You can't beat the convenience of canned tuna but let's face it, tuna sandwiches can get a bit boring after a while. For a change of pace, try these Corny Tuna Cakes. They're as easy to make as pancakes and we promise your kids will compliment your cooking when they taste them. The inspiration for this recipe came from crab cakes. But rather than use regular mayonnaise and ½ stick of butter to fry them, we lightened things up a bit.

Moms Make It Over By . . .

- Adding corn for vitamins, minerals, phytonutrients, and fiber.
- Using light canola mayonnaise and cooking in a moderate amount of healthy canola oil to lower the saturated fat and calories.

> **Two 6-ounce cans solid white, water-packed tuna, drained and flaked**
>
> **¾ cup preshredded reduced-fat Cheddar cheese**
>
> **¾ cup dried bread crumbs, divided**
>
> **⅔ cup frozen corn kernels, thawed**
>
> **⅓ cup light canola mayonnaise**
>
> **1 large egg, beaten**
>
> **1 tablespoon canola oil**

1. Combine the tuna, cheese, ¼ cup bread crumbs, the corn, mayonnaise, and egg in a medium bowl and mix until well blended.

2. Shape the mixture into 8 patties and coat with the remaining ½ cup bread crumbs.

3. Heat half the oil in a large nonstick skillet over medium heat. Cook the patties until golden brown, about 5 minutes. Add the remaining oil to the skillet, flip the patties, and cook an additional 4 to 5 minutes.

PREPARATION TIME: 15 MINUTES
COOKING TIME: 10 MINUTES

	Before	After
Calories	550	340
Fat (g)	33	14
Saturated Fat (g)	13	2.5
Sodium (mg)	1,270	740
Carbohydrate (g)	31	22
Fiber (g)	1	1
Protein (g)	31	30

Moms' Kitchen Notes: For a bigger omega-3 boost, use two 6-ounce cans of skinless, boneless pink salmon.

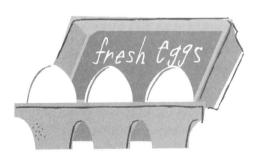

Linguine with Clam Sauce

MAKES 4 SERVINGS

Janice has a neighbor who swears by her linguine with clam sauce, claiming that even her grand-children love it. We were intrigued, since most kids don't usually ask for this sort of dish. Grandma's recipe really sounded delicious but to our disappointment, the amount of sodium rivaled that found in seawater. Here's why: It turns out that canned minced clams and white clam sauce are often loaded with salt (not to mention monosodium glutamate in the latter).

Moms Make It Over By . . .

- Adding asparagus for vitamins, minerals, phytonutrients, and fiber.
- Using minced clams and less clam juice to lower the sodium.
- Using 2 ounces of dried pasta per serving to keep the portions and calories in check.

 8 ounces dried linguine

 1 tablespoon olive oil

 1 teaspoon bottled crushed garlic, or 1 to 2 garlic cloves, minced

 8 ounces asparagus, trimmed and cut into ½-inch pieces

 One 14½-ounce can diced tomatoes

 ¾ cup 1% lowfat milk

 2 tablespoons all-purpose flour

 One 6½-ounce can minced clams, drained

 One 6½-ounce can minced clams, undrained

 ¼ cup grated Parmesan cheese

1. Cook the pasta according to package directions. Drain and return to the pan.

2. While the pasta is cooking, heat the oil in a large nonstick skillet over medium heat. Add the garlic and asparagus and cook, stirring frequently, 1 to 2 minutes.

3. Add the tomatoes, raise the heat, and bring to a boil. Reduce the heat and simmer until the asparagus softens, about 10 minutes.

4. Combine the milk and flour in a bowl and whisk until well blended. Add the milk mixture, 1 can of drained clams, and 1 can of undrained clams to the skillet.

5. Bring to a simmer, stirring constantly. Reduce the heat and continue to simmer and stir gently until the mixture thickens slightly, about 2 minutes.

6. Pour the sauce over the linguine and toss to combine. Serve in individual bowls and sprinkle with Parmesan cheese.

PREPARATION TIME: **10 MINUTES**
COOKING TIME: **20 MINUTES**

	Before	After
Calories	540	360
Fat (g)	24	7
Saturated Fat (g)	5	2
Sodium (mg)	1,550	570
Carbohydrate (g)	60	57
Fiber (g)	3	4
Protein (g)	22	21

Moms' Kitchen Notes: If your kids are particular about the texture of cooked vegetables and prefer them soft, cook the asparagus for a few extra minutes.

Seafood: Superstar of Land and Sea

Seafood's health benefits come in part from its omega-3 fatty acids. While it often surprises people to hear that fat is actually good for them, research shows that omega-3s may lower the risk of heart disease and reduce the symptoms of rheumatoid arthritis and depression. Unfortunately, on average, Americans only get about 15 percent of the omega-3s they need each day. So the big question is . . . how much do we need? Well, in the United States, there is no official recommended daily intake but some health experts suggest a minimum of ½ to 1 gram (500 milligrams to 1,000 milligrams) a day. Check out the chart below to discover how seafood can increase your family's omega-3 intake.

SEAFOOD	GRAMS OF OMEGA-3 FATS PER 4 OUNCES COOKED
Salmon, Atlantic	2.2
Sardines, in tomato sauce	1.9
Oysters	1.5
Trout	1.3
Mackerel, canned	1.3
Tuna, white, canned in water	0.9
Flounder or Sole	0.6
Shrimp	0.4
Catfish	0.3
Clams	0.2

Grilled Salmon with Ginger Honey Glaze

MAKES 4 SERVINGS

It's hard to enjoy a meal when the kids are whining that they want something else. If you grew up eating plain broiled fish with a squeeze of lemon you'll know what we mean. The way Janice keeps the complaints at bay at her house is to serve her dad's Grilled Salmon with Ginger Honey Glaze.

Moms Make It Over By . . .

- Creating a glaze with honey, ginger, and teriyaki to pump up the flavor.
- Using salmon to increase the healthy omega-3 fats.

> 1¼ pounds salmon fillet with skin
>
> Salt and pepper
>
> 2 tablespoons lite teriyaki sauce
>
> 1 tablespoon honey
>
> 2 tablespoons bottled minced ginger, or 1 teaspoon ground ginger

1. Preheat the grill on high heat.

2. Season the salmon with salt and pepper.

3. Combine the teriyaki sauce and honey and pour evenly over the salmon. Spread the ginger over the top. Let sit for 5 to 10 minutes while the grill is heating.

4. Place the salmon, skin side up, on the grill and cook 5 minutes over high heat. Turn gently, reduce the heat to medium, and grill until the salmon is cooked through and flakes easily with a fork, 7 to 10 minutes. Remove the skin and serve.

PREPARATION TIME: 5 MINUTES
COOKING TIME: 15 MINUTES

	Before	After
Calories	100	250
Fat (g)	1	10
Saturated Fat (g)	0	1.5
Sodium (mg)	75	230
Carbohydrate (g)	0	6
Fiber (g)	0	0
Protein (g)	22	33

Moms' Kitchen Notes: Serve with grilled vegetables such as zucchini, asparagus, Portobello mushrooms, or eggplant.

Walnut-Crusted Salmon

MAKES 4 SERVINGS

For a lot of people, ordering a seafood dinner means a meal of fried fish & chips or perhaps a simple piece of baked white fish topped with a mixture of cracker crumbs and butter. Well, it's time to rethink your "catch of the day." If you're looking to get hooked on something new, choose salmon, the king of the sea when it comes to healthy omega-3 fats. For a double dose, we created a delicious topping with walnuts . . . another source of omega-3s.

Moms Make It Over By . . .

🥕 Creating a topping with walnuts and bread crumbs instead of cracker crumbs and butter to lower the saturated fat and increase the healthy omega-3 fats.

½ cup walnuts, finely chopped

2 tablespoons dried bread crumbs

1 tablespoon all-fruit apricot jam

1 tablespoon balsamic vinegar

1¼ pounds salmon fillet, skinned

Salt and pepper

1. Preheat the oven to 400°F.

2. Combine the walnuts and bread crumbs, arrange on a plate, and set aside.

3. Mix together the jam and vinegar in a small bowl.

4. Season the salmon with salt and pepper. Brush both sides with the jam mixture. Coat both sides evenly with the walnut mixture, pressing the extra breading evenly over the top.

5. Place in a baking pan and bake until the fish is cooked through and flakes easily with a fork, 15 to 20 minutes, depending on the thickness of the salmon.

PREPARATION TIME: **10 MINUTES**
COOKING TIME: **15 TO 20 MINUTES**

Moms' Kitchen Notes: Don't forget to ask the person behind the seafood counter to skin the salmon fillet for you.

	Before	After
Calories	230	360
Fat (g)	10	20
Saturated Fat (g)	6	2.5
Sodium (mg)	360	180
Carbohydrate (g)	12	8
Fiber (g)	<1	1
Protein (g)	20	35

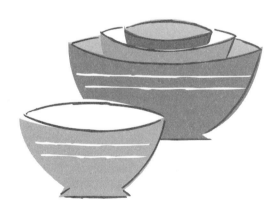

Shrimp Curry in a Hurry

MAKES 4 TO 5 SERVINGS

When a dish calls for cream, egg yolks, and butter, you automatically think of a rich and decadent dessert. But believe it or not, these are also the ingredients used in shrimp Newberg. This extraordinarily rich dish really takes the cake with its 30-plus grams of fat in a serving. Our very simple makeover gets the fat down and the vegetables up.

Moms Make It Over By . . .

🍓 Adding broccoli for vitamins, minerals, phytonutrients, and fiber.

🍓 Creating a sauce with lowfat milk and reduced-fat sour cream to lower the saturated fat and calories.

> 4 cups fresh or frozen broccoli florets
>
> 2 cups instant brown rice (about 4 cups cooked)
>
> 1 tablespoon olive oil
>
> 1 small onion, finely chopped (about ½ cup)
>
> 1½ to 2 teaspoons curry powder
>
> 1 teaspoon garlic powder
>
> ½ teaspoon salt
>
> 1½ cups 1% lowfat milk
>
> 3 tablespoons all-purpose flour
>
> 1 pound small or medium cooked shrimp, fresh or frozen, thawed
>
> ½ cup reduced-fat sour cream
>
> ¼ cup roasted cashews, optional

1. Steam the broccoli until tender, about 5 minutes. Remove from the heat and set aside uncovered.

2. Cook the rice according to package directions.

3. While the rice is cooking, heat the oil in a large nonstick skillet over medium-high heat. Add the onion, curry powder, garlic powder, and salt and cook, stirring frequently, until the onion is translucent, 5 to 7 minutes.

4. Meanwhile, whisk together the milk and flour in a bowl until well blended.

5. Add the milk mixture, broccoli, and shrimp to the skillet and bring to a simmer, stirring constantly. Reduce the heat and continue to simmer and stir gently until the liquid thickens slightly, about 2 minutes.

6. Add the sour cream and heat through. Serve over rice and sprinkle with cashews as desired.

PREPARATION TIME: 15 MINUTES
COOKING TIME: 15 MINUTES

	Before	After
Calories	550	400
Fat (g)	33	10
Saturated Fat (g)	14	3
Sodium (mg)	650	570
Carbohydrate (g)	30	51
Fiber (g)	2	4
Protein (g)	20	31

Moms' Kitchen Notes: Be careful not to overcook the broccoli. If you do, it may end up falling apart and turning the sauce green!

Sweet & Slightly Sour Shrimp

MAKES 5 SERVINGS

Sweet & sour shrimp sounds so innocent, and in theory it should be. But in many restaurants, this popular dish is often breaded, deep fried, and then smothered in a gooey sweet and salty sauce. Even before you toss it over rice, sweet & sour shrimp can have over 500 calories and a teaspoon's worth of sodium in a serving. Our made-over version is just as appealing, but a whole lot lighter.

Moms Make It Over By . . .

- Adding mixed vegetables for vitamins, minerals, phytonutrients, and fiber.
- Cooking in a moderate amount of peanut oil to lower the saturated fat and calories.
- Using lite teriyaki sauce to lower the sodium.

> 2 cups instant brown rice (about 4 cups cooked)
>
> One 8-ounce can pineapple tidbits or chunks packed in juice
>
> ⅓ cup water or all-natural chicken broth
>
> ⅓ cup lite teriyaki sauce
>
> 2 tablespoons white wine vinegar or rice vinegar
>
> 2 tablespoons all-natural peanut butter, optional
>
> 2 tablespoons cornstarch
>
> 1 tablespoon peanut oil
>
> One 16-ounce bag frozen Asian-style mixed vegetables, thawed
>
> ½ teaspoon ground ginger, or 1 teaspoon bottled minced ginger
>
> 1 pound small or medium cooked shrimp, fresh or frozen, thawed

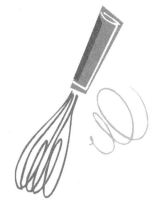

1. Cook the rice according to package directions. Set aside.

2. Drain the juice from the pineapple into a bowl. Set the pineapple aside. To the pineapple juice, add the water, teriyaki sauce, vinegar, peanut butter as desired, and cornstarch and whisk until well blended. Set aside.

3. Heat the oil in a large nonstick skillet or wok over high heat, add the vegetables and ginger, and stir-fry for 3 minutes.

4. Add the shrimp and pineapple and cook, stirring frequently, until heated through, 1 to 2 minutes.

5. Rewhisk the pineapple juice mixture and add to the skillet. Bring to a simmer, stirring constantly. Reduce the heat and continue to simmer and stir gently until the mixture thickens slightly, about 2 minutes.

6. Serve over the rice.

PREPARATION TIME: 10 MINUTES
COOKING TIME: 15 MINUTES

	Before	After
Calories	480	320
Fat (g)	30	5
Saturated Fat (g)	4	0
Sodium (mg)	2,020	610
Carbohydrate (g)	46	46
Fiber (g)	1	3
Protein (g)	12	25

Moms' Kitchen Notes: If you can't find frozen Asian vegetables, use a bag of any other frozen mixed vegetables that your family likes.

Shrimp "Not-So-Fried" Rice

MAKES 4 TO 5 SERVINGS

We never miss an opportunity to transform a recipe from nutritionally average to awesome. That was recently the case with a recipe for fried rice given to us by a busy mom in need of new strategies for getting her kids to eat more vegetables. Her recipe was garnished with only a handful of bean sprouts . . . which to her frustration, the kids always picked out.

Moms Make It Over By . . .

- Adding mixed vegetables for vitamins, minerals, phytonutrients, and fiber.
- Including shrimp for lean protein and healthy omega-3 fats.

2 tablespoons lite soy sauce

3 tablespoons hoisin sauce

1 teaspoon garlic powder

½ teaspoon ground ginger, or 1 teaspoon bottled minced ginger

2 large eggs

1 tablespoon toasted sesame oil

3 green onions and tops, minced, optional

1 pound small or medium cooked shrimp, fresh or frozen, thawed

One 16-ounce bag frozen mixed vegetables, thawed

2 cups chilled cooked jasmine or basmati rice

1. Combine the soy sauce, hoisin sauce, garlic powder, and ginger in a small bowl and mix well. Set aside.

2. Beat the eggs with 2 tablespoons water until blended.

3. Heat the oil in a large nonstick skillet or wok over medium-high heat. Add the green onions if desired and stir-fry 1 minute. Add the eggs and stir-fry to a soft scramble, 30 seconds.

4. Add the shrimp, vegetables, and soy sauce mixture and cook on high heat, stirring frequently, until heated through, 3 minutes.

5. Stir in the rice and cook until hot, about 3 minutes.

PREPARATION TIME: 15 MINUTES
COOKING TIME: 10 MINUTES

Moms' Kitchen Notes: If your children prefer their vegetables very soft, add them to the skillet before the eggs and cook 2 to 3 minutes. Also, be sure to cook your rice ahead of time because it needs to be chilled for this recipe.

	Before	After
Calories	380	350
Fat (g)	21	7
Saturated Fat (g)	3.5	1
Sodium (mg)	990	750
Carbohydrate (g)	36	41
Fiber (g)	1	3
Protein (g)	14	29

Almond Battered Fish

MAKES 6 SERVINGS

Fish is usually a healthy meal option but once a fast food restaurant gets its hands on it . . . all bets are off. The idea for this recipe makeover came from a fast food fried fish sandwich. The amount of refined carbs in the sandwich (i.e., the breading and the bun) was three times higher than the protein (i.e., the fish). We also discovered a few grams of artery-clogging trans fats in the dish, something you'll often find in fast food items that have been fried.

Moms Make It Over By . . .

- Cooking in a moderate amount of healthy canola oil to lower the saturated fat and eliminate the trans fats.
- Using whole wheat flour in the batter for added nutrients and fiber.
- Including almonds in the batter for added nutrients and heart-healthy monounsaturated fats.

> $2/3$ cup slivered almonds, very finely chopped
>
> $1/2$ cup all-purpose flour
>
> $1/3$ cup whole wheat flour
>
> $3/4$ teaspoon salt
>
> $1/4$ teaspoon baking powder
>
> 1 cup 1% lowfat milk
>
> 3 tablespoons canola oil
>
> 6 fresh or frozen fish fillets such as flounder, trout, or tilapia, thawed if frozen (about $1/2$ pounds)
>
> Tartar sauce, for serving (see Moms' Kitchen Notes, below)

1. Whisk together the almonds, all-purpose flour, whole wheat flour, salt, and baking powder in a large bowl. Add the milk and whisk until smooth.

2. Heat half the oil in a large nonstick skillet over medium-high heat.

3. Working in batches, dip the fish into the batter, coating evenly on all sides. Place half the fish into the skillet and cook until golden brown, 3 to 4 minutes per side depending on the thickness of the fish. Repeat with the remaining oil and fish. Adjust the heat if necessary.

4. Serve with tartar sauce.

PREPARATION TIME: 15 MINUTES
COOKING TIME: 15 MINUTES

	Before	After
Calories	470	320
Fat (g)	26	16
Saturated Fat (g)	5	1.5
Sodium (mg)	730	440
Carbohydrate (g)	45	18
Fiber (g)	1	2
Protein (g)	15	25

Moms' Kitchen Notes: To make your own tartar sauce, mix together ⅓ cup light canola mayonnaise, 2 tablespoons relish, 1 tablespoon ketchup, and 1 teaspoon bottled or fresh lemon juice.

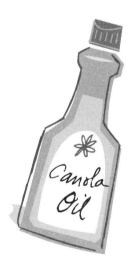

Baked Fish with Spinach Cheese Sauce

MAKES 6 SERVINGS

When the word "Florentine" is used to describe a dish, it means there's spinach somewhere in the recipe. That's the case with seafood Florentine, where the fish is layered with creamed spinach, a white sauce, butter, and bread crumbs. The result can be nearly a day's worth of saturated fat in a serving. Using a few culinary tools and tricks, we renovated this flavorful recipe and reeled in most of the unhealthy fat.

Moms Make It Over By . . .

🫀 Creating a sauce with lowfat milk and reduced-fat cheese to lower the saturated fat and calories.

🫀 Using less added salt to reduce the sodium.

 ½ cup dried bread crumbs

 ¼ cup plus 2 tablespoons grated Parmesan cheese

 ¼ teaspoon garlic powder

 ¼ teaspoon onion powder

 Pinch of pepper

 3 tablespoons olive oil or canola oil, divided

 2 pounds cod, haddock, or other firm white fish, cut into 6 pieces

 One 6-ounce package prewashed baby spinach (about 4 packed cups)

 1½ cups 1% lowfat milk

 3 tablespoons all-purpose flour

 Pinch of ground nutmeg

 1 cup preshredded reduced-fat Cheddar cheese

1. Preheat the oven to 450°F.

2. Combine the bread crumbs, ¼ cup of the Parmesan cheese, the garlic powder, onion powder, and pepper in a shallow bowl. Place 2 tablespoons of the oil in a separate bowl. Lightly coat each piece of fish in the oil, then coat evenly with the bread crumb mixture.

3. Arrange the fish on a baking sheet and cook until the fish is cooked through and flakes easily with a fork, about 15 minutes, depending on the thickness.

4. Meanwhile, heat the remaining tablespoon of oil in a medium saucepan over medium-high heat.

Add the spinach and cook, stirring frequently, until the spinach wilts and is fully cooked, 4 to 5 minutes.

5. While the spinach is cooking, whisk together the milk, flour, and nutmeg in a bowl until well blended. When the spinach is done, add the milk mixture to the saucepan and bring to a simmer, stirring constantly. Reduce the heat and continue to simmer and stir gently until the mixture thickens slightly, about 2 minutes.

6. Stir in the Cheddar cheese and the remaining 2 tablespoons Parmesan cheese until melted.

7. Place the fish on individual plates. Pour the sauce over each piece and serve.

PREPARATION TIME: 20 MINUTES
COOKING TIME: 20 MINUTES

	Before	After
Calories	510	310
Fat (g)	31	12
Saturated Fat (g)	18	3.5
Sodium (mg)	1,080	420
Carbohydrate (g)	18	14
Fiber (g)	2	2
Protein (g)	39	35

Moms' Kitchen Notes: Serve over whole wheat couscous or rice.

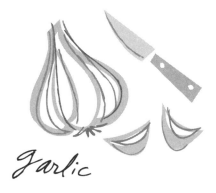

Garlic

Cheesy Pecan Fish Rolls

MAKES 4 SERVINGS

The next time you're fishing for a compliment at the dinner table, you must, must, try this recipe handed down from Janice's mom. We guarantee there will be no eye rolling when this dish hits the table. Instead of the usual stuffed seafood dish made with a buttery filling of cracker crumbs and a few gratuitous bits of celery, the "breading" turns this dish inside out!

Moms Make It Over By . . .

- Stuffing the fish with reduced-fat cheese to lower the saturated fat and calories.
- Coating the fish with pecans for added nutrients and heart-healthy mono-unsaturated fats.

> ½ cup pecans, finely chopped
> ¼ cup dried bread crumbs
> 2 to 3 tablespoons canola oil
> 1¼ pounds thin fish fillets, such as sole or flounder (approximately 6 to 10 small fillets)
> Salt and pepper
> 3 ounces reduced-fat Swiss cheese, thinly sliced

1. Preheat the oven to 400°F.
2. Lightly oil or coat a 9 x 13-inch baking pan with nonstick cooking spray and set aside.
3. Combine the pecans and bread crumbs in a small bowl and set aside. Place the oil in a separate bowl.
4. Lay the fillets on a cutting board or work surface and season with salt and pepper.
5. Cut the cheese into strips to match the size of the fillets and place a slice on top of each. Roll up the fish starting with the thin end.
6. Carefully dip the fish in the oil, then coat evenly with the pecan mixture.
7. Arrange the rolls, seam side down, on the prepared baking pan. Bake until the coating turns

golden brown, the cheese melts, and the fish is cooked through, 15 to 25 minutes, depending on the thickness of the fillets.

PREPARATION TIME: 15 MINUTES
COOKING TIME: 15 TO 25 MINUTES

Moms' Kitchen Notes: If the fillets are more than 3 or 4 inches wide, slice them lengthwise down the middle to create two smaller pieces.

	Before	After
Calories	500	340
Fat (g)	30	21
Saturated Fat (g)	16	2.5
Sodium (mg)	1,410	220
Carbohydrate (g)	13	8
Fiber (g)	<1	2
Protein (g)	43	32

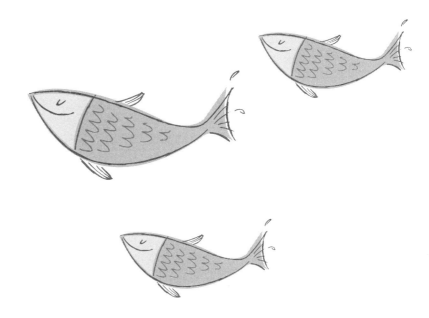

Shrimp and Cholesterol: Myth or Reality?

If you think eating shrimp is a no-no for people watching their cholesterol, there's no need to flounder anymore. A 3-ounce portion of shrimp contains about half of the recommended daily intake of cholesterol. And since it doesn't contain any saturated fat, shrimp is a smart choice at the seafood counter. The caveat here is that drowning shrimp or other shellfish in butter and heavy cream sauces can send the fat and cholesterol soaring. So be mindful of how you prepare your favorite shellfish to take advantage of its best qualities.

MAKING SENSE OF SHELLFISH
3-OUNCE PORTION

	CALORIES	TOTAL FAT (GRAMS)	SATURATED FAT (GRAMS)	CHOLESTEROL (MILLIGRAMS)
Shrimp	81	1	0	167
Crab	101	1	0	91
Lobster	83	0.5	0.9	61
Clams	126	1.5	0.2	57
Scallops	114	3	0.6	34

CHAPTER 12

Perfect Poultry

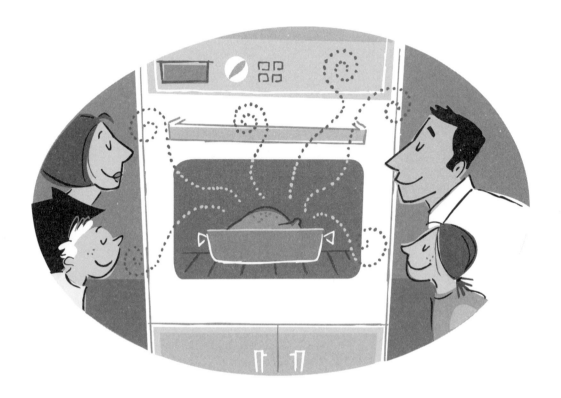

Krispy Honey-Fried Drumsticks • No-Nonsense Nuggets • Confetti Chicken Wraps • Cheesy Chicken Divan • Moroccan Un-Stuffed Peppers • Oh-So-Easy Chicken Parmesan • Colorful Cacciatore • Fit 'n Trim Tetrazzini • Southwestern Chicken & Rice • "Mom, the House Smells Great" Roasted Chicken • Turkey Meat Loaf Muffins • Jolly Green Bean & Chicken Casserole

There's no doubt that we're a nation of meat-and-potato lovers, but it's clear that Americans are also crazy about chicken. Over the past two decades alone, people on average have increased their yearly chicken consumption from 33 pounds to 53 pounds per person. The reasons for chicken's rise in the pecking order are many including cost, nutrition, taste, and ease of preparation.

A 3-ounce portion of baked skinless chicken breast has just 140 calories and 3 grams of fat. But while chicken may start out lean, busy families often flock to fried chicken, fast food chicken sandwiches, and chicken nuggets, which ups the fat content significantly. For that reason, plus a few more, we felt a chicken makeover was in order.

One of our favorite recipes is No-Nonsense Nuggets (page 276), a simple renovation for the chicken nuggets most kids like to eat. Our revamped recipe has just 7 grams of fat, a far cry from the 20-plus grams found in some of the more popular frozen and fast food brands. But perhaps more important, our nuggets are also a lot higher in protein—a nutrient active children need for normal growth. Since we use skinless, boneless chicken breast meat instead of those mysterious spongelike chicken pieces, our meal is the real deal. Another big favorite is our "Mom, the House Smells Great" Roasted Chicken (page 294), bursting with flavor and cooked to perfection (not cardboard). Your kids will love coming home to this one.

The next time your family whines "Oh no, not chicken again," try these twelve dynamite dishes, and the complaints may just turn into compliments.

Krispy Honey-Fried Drumsticks

MAKES 5 TO 6 SERVINGS

How many napkins do you go through when you eat fried chicken? A dozen? Two dozen? While nothing could be more all-American than fried chicken, it can be downright greasy. Our easy makeover uses honey and teriyaki sauce instead of the usual inch or two of oil for a dinner that's finger-licking good.

Moms Make It Over By ...

- Using skinless drumsticks and baking instead of frying to lower the total fat, saturated fat, and calories.
- Using lite teriyaki and only a small amount of added salt to reduce the sodium.

> **2 cups Rice Krispies cereal**
>
> **½ cup pecans, finely chopped**
>
> **3 tablespoons honey**
>
> **2 tablespoons lite teriyaki sauce**
>
> **12 drumsticks, skinned (about 3 pounds)**
>
> **Salt and pepper**

1. Preheat the oven to 425°F.

2. Place the Rice Krispies in a bowl and crush slightly with your hands. Stir in the pecans and set aside.

3. Place the honey and teriyaki sauce in a large bowl and stir to combine.

4. Season the chicken with salt and pepper. Place drumsticks in the honey mixture and toss to coat evenly. Working with one drumstick at a time, roll in the cereal mixture until well coated (lay it on thick).

5. Place the chicken on a large baking sheet and cook until the meat is done and the coating turns golden brown, about 30 minutes.

PREPARATION TIME: 15 TO 20 MINUTES

COOKING TIME: 30 MINUTES

	Before	After
Calories	750	350
Fat (g)	45	15
Saturated Fat (g)	12	2.5
Sodium (mg)	1,070	250
Carbohydrate (g)	26	22
Fiber (g)	0	1
Protein (g)	55	32

No-Nonsense Nuggets

MAKES 4 SERVINGS

Chicken nuggets are perfect when you're in a pinch, but a lot of the frozen brands out there are made with processed chicken and a thick layer of greasy breading. With our No-Nonsense Nuggets, you know exactly what you're getting. Serve them with ketchup and don't feel guilty because ketchup contains lycopene, an antioxidant that may ward off heart disease and certain cancers.

Moms Make It Over By . . .

- Using skinless, boneless chicken breast to lower the saturated fat and increase the protein.
- Baking instead of frying.

> 3 cups corn flakes
>
> ⅓ cup grated Parmesan cheese
>
> ½ teaspoon salt
>
> ¼ teaspoon onion powder
>
> ¼ teaspoon garlic powder
>
> Pinch of pepper
>
> 1 pound skinless, boneless chicken breast halves, cut into nugget-size pieces
>
> ¼ cup all-purpose flour
>
> 2 large eggs, beaten

1. Preheat the oven to 425°F.

2. Lightly oil or coat a large baking sheet with nonstick cooking spray and set aside.

3. Place the corn flakes in a resealable plastic bag and crush to a fine texture using a rolling pin or the bottom of a small saucepan, or place in a food processor and pulse several turns until finely crushed. Combine with the Parmesan cheese, salt, onion powder, garlic powder, and pepper in a medium bowl.

4. To bread the chicken, coat in flour, shaking off excess. Dip in the egg, then coat well in the corn flake mixture.

5. Arrange the chicken on the prepared baking sheet and cook until golden brown, about 12 minutes.

PREPARATION TIME: 20 MINUTES
COOKING TIME: 15 MINUTES

	Before	After
Calories	290	290
Fat (g)	21	7
Saturated Fat (g)	5	3
Sodium (mg)	470	510
Carbohydrate (g)	15	25
Fiber (g)	1	1
Protein (g)	10	31

Moms' Kitchen Notes: Serve with Sweet Potato Fries (page 304).

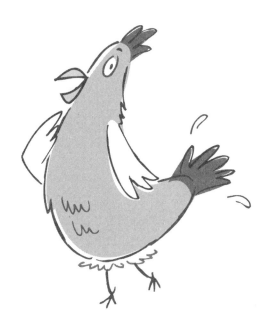

Confetti Chicken Wraps

MAKES 6 TO 8 SERVINGS

What do orange bell peppers and yellow corn kernels have in common? Yes, yes, we know they're both vegetables, but it turns out that each contains a powerful antioxidant called zeaxanthin. Research suggests that zeaxanthin keeps our eyes healthy as we age. Besides the fact that orange peppers and corn are good for you, they also taste great in this simple weeknight meal. You may never turn to fast food tacos or burritos again after you try our wraps.

Moms Make It Over By . . .

🍓 Adding bell pepper and corn for vitamins, minerals, phytonutrients, and fiber.

🍓 Using skinless, boneless chicken breast to lower the saturated fat.

1 tablespoon canola oil

1 large orange bell pepper, diced or cut into thin, 1-inch strips (about 1 ½ cups)

1 pound skinless, boneless chicken breast halves, sliced into thin strips

½ to 1 teaspoon ground cumin

½ to 1 teaspoon chili powder

One 15½-ounce can pinto beans, drained and rinsed

1 cup frozen corn kernels, thawed

1 cup preshredded reduced-fat Cheddar cheese

¾ cup salsa

Six to eight 8-inch flour tortillas

½ cup reduced-fat sour cream, optional

1. Heat the oil in a large nonstick skillet over medium-high heat. Add the bell pepper and cook, stirring frequently, until tender, about 5 minutes.

2. Add the chicken, cumin, and chili powder and cook until the chicken is no longer pink, 4 to 5 minutes.

3. Stir in the beans, corn, cheese, and salsa and cook until heated through and the cheese melts, about 2 minutes.

4. Meanwhile, stack the tortillas on a microwave-safe plate, uncovered, and heat in the microwave until warmed through, 30 to 45 seconds.

5. Assemble by placing the chicken mixture down the center of each tortilla. Wrap burrito-style and serve with sour cream as desired.

PREPARATION TIME: **15 MINUTES**
COOKING TIME: **15 MINUTES**

	Before	After
Calories	390	330
Fat (g)	16	8
Saturated Fat (g)	6	1.5
Sodium (mg)	930	510
Carbohydrate (g)	41	41
Fiber (g)	7	8
Protein (g)	21	24

Moms' Kitchen Notes: Kick up the flavor by using a medium or hot salsa or by increasing the amount of cumin and chili powder.

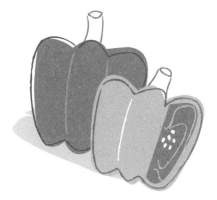

Home Food Safety: It's in Your Hands

Chicken and turkey can carry salmonella and other harmful bacteria that may cause food poisoning. We're not trying to ruin your appetite, but when poultry (or any raw meat) is on your dinner menu, be sure to follow these four simple food safety guidelines.

POULTRY POINTER #1: WASH YOUR HANDS

Wash your hands in hot or warm soapy water before and after food preparation and make sure you do it for 20 seconds. Actually, count to 20 the next time you're at the sink, because what you've been doing may be closer to a quick rinse.

POULTRY POINTER #2: KEEP RAW MEATS AND READY-TO-EAT FOODS SEPARATE

If the juices from raw poultry or meat come in contact with the ingredients for your dinner salad, there could be trouble at the table. To prevent cross-contamination, keep two plastic cutting boards in your kitchen—one for raw meats and the other for ready-to-eat foods like vegetables and bread. Also, during grilling season, remember that cooked chicken should never go back on the same plate that held the raw chicken.

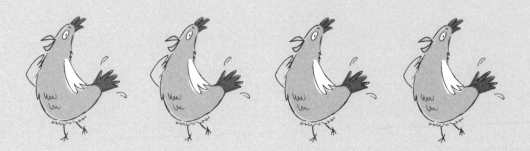

POULTRY POINTER #3: COOK TO PROPER TEMPERATURES

Dangerous bacteria are killed when food is cooked to the proper temperature. While seasoned chefs and some savvy home cooks can tell if meat is done by simply poking it, most of us are better off buying an inexpensive instant-read meat thermometer . . . and using it. To be on the safe side, stick with the following "safe cooking temperatures" for poultry and other meats:

Boneless chicken and turkey breast	170°F
Whole chicken and turkey, thighs, wings, and drumsticks	180°F
Hamburgers	160°F
Steak, medium-rare	145°F

POULTRY POINTER #4: REFRIGERATE PROMPTLY BELOW 40°F

Ask ten people what the temperature of their refrigerator should be and chances are you'll get ten different answers. Is it 30°F, 55°F, 20°F? The answer is below 40°F. Bacteria love to grow between 40°F and 140°F, so if the temperature inside your fridge is above 40°F, bad bacteria can have a field day.

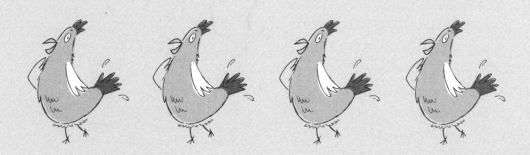

Cheesy Chicken Divan

MAKES 4 SERVINGS

A lot of the health-conscious moms that we know have shied away from all those fun classic casseroles from the fifties and sixties because they're often loaded with butter and cream. So when a friend asked us to give her favorite chicken divan recipe a face-lift, we took on the challenge, creating a dish with less fat and more flavor than ever before.

Moms Make It Over By . . .

- Using lowfat milk and reduced-fat cheese to lower the saturated fat and increase the bone-building calcium.

One 10-ounce box frozen chopped broccoli

½ cup dried bread crumbs

5 tablespoons grated Parmesan cheese, divided

½ teaspoon dried tarragon

½ teaspoon garlic powder

¼ teaspoon salt

1 to 2 tablespoons olive oil

1 pound thin-sliced skinless, boneless chicken breast cutlets

1½ cups 1% lowfat milk

2 tablespoons all-purpose flour

½ teaspoon Dijon mustard

1 cup preshredded reduced-fat Cheddar cheese

2 tablespoons grated Parmesan cheese

1. Preheat the oven to 425°F.

2. Cook the broccoli according to package directions. Cover and set aside.

3. Combine the bread crumbs, 3 tablespoons Parmesan cheese, tarragon, garlic powder, and salt in a shallow bowl. Place the oil in a separate bowl. Lightly coat each chicken cutlet with the oil, then coat evenly with the bread crumb mixture.

4. Arrange the chicken on a large baking sheet and bake until the meat is no longer pink, 12 to 14 minutes.

5. While the chicken is cooking, whisk together the milk, flour, and Dijon mustard in a medium saucepan until well blended. Place over medium-high heat and bring to a simmer, stirring constantly. Reduce the heat and continue to simmer and stir gently until the mixture thickens slightly, about 2 minutes. Stir in the Cheddar cheese and 2 tablespoons Parmesan cheese and cook until melted. Stir in the broccoli.

6. Place the chicken on individual plates. Pour the sauce over each cutlet and serve.

PREPARATION TIME: 15 MINUTES
COOKING TIME: 15 MINUTES

	Before	After
Calories	350	350
Fat (g)	22	12
Saturated Fat (g)	13	4.5
Sodium (mg)	770	690
Carbohydrate (g)	10	21
Fiber (g)	3	3
Protein (g)	27	39

Moms' Kitchen Notes: If you can't find thin-sliced chicken cutlets, make your own by placing skinless, boneless chicken breast halves between two sheets of plastic wrap or wax paper. Using a meat mallet or the bottom of a small saucepan, flatten to ¼-inch thickness.

Moroccan Un-Stuffed Peppers

MAKES 6 SERVINGS

If the stuffed green peppers of your youth were made with a mixture of fatty ground beef, onions, and rice, we think you'll welcome our more flavorful and healthful makeover. Moroccan Un-Stuffed Peppers go out of the box with raisins, almonds, and couscous . . . not to mention peppers that don't need to be stuffed!

Moms Make It Over By . . .

- Adding carrots and raisins for vitamins, minerals, phytonutrients, and fiber.
- Switching to lean ground turkey to lower the saturated fat.
- Including almonds for added nutrients and heart-healthy monounsaturated fats.

> 8 ounces whole wheat couscous (about 1⅓ cups)
>
> 1 tablespoon canola oil
>
> 1¼ pounds lean ground turkey
>
> 3 cups frozen bell pepper strips or 2 medium red or yellow bell peppers, finely diced (about 2 cups)
>
> 1 cup preshredded carrots or 1 large carrot, shredded (about 1 cup)
>
> ½ cup golden raisins
>
> 2 teaspoons ground cumin
>
> 1 teaspoon onion powder
>
> 1 teaspoon ground cinnamon
>
> ¾ teaspoon salt
>
> 1½ cups all-natural chicken broth
>
> 2 tablespoons all-purpose flour
>
> ⅓ cup slivered almonds

1. Cook the couscous according to package directions and set aside.
2. Heat the oil in a large nonstick skillet or Dutch oven over medium-high heat. Add the turkey,

bell peppers, carrots, raisins, cumin, onion powder, cinnamon, and salt and cook, breaking up the large pieces of turkey, until the vegetables are tender and the meat is no longer pink, 5 to 7 minutes.

3. Meanwhile, whisk together the broth and flour in a small bowl. Add to the turkey mixture and stir until the liquid thickens, about 2 minutes.

4. Serve in individual bowls over couscous and top with almonds.

PREPARATION TIME: 15 MINUTES
COOKING TIME: 10 MINUTES

	Before	After
Calories	380	430
Fat (g)	16	15
Saturated Fat (g)	7	2.5
Sodium (mg)	910	540
Carbohydrate (g)	40	51
Fiber (g)	4	9
Protein (g)	20	25

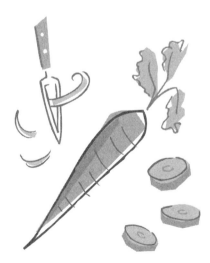

Oh-So-Easy Chicken Parmesan

MAKES 5 SERVINGS

Our children tend to order chicken Parmesan whenever we eat Italian . . . and why not? The flavor is hard to resist. But depending on how it's prepared, chicken Parmesan can be loaded with fat and sodium. Traditional recipes often call for lots of oil and a hefty layer of full-fat cheese. But not ours.

Moms Make It Over By . . .

- Using part-skim cheese and a moderate amount of healthy olive oil to lower the saturated fat and calories.
- Adding less salt to reduce the sodium.

½ cup dried bread crumbs

¼ cup grated Parmesan cheese

½ teaspoon garlic powder

¼ teaspoon salt

1 to 2 tablespoons olive oil

1¼ pounds thin-sliced skinless, boneless chicken breast cutlets

1 cup pasta sauce

1 cup preshredded part-skim mozzarella cheese

1. Preheat the oven to 425°F.

2. Combine the bread crumbs, Parmesan cheese, garlic powder, and salt in a shallow bowl. Place the olive oil in a separate bowl. Lightly coat each cutlet with the oil then coat evenly with the bread crumb mixture.

3. Arrange the chicken on a large baking sheet and bake until the meat is no longer pink, 12 to 14 minutes.

4. Pour the pasta sauce evenly over the chicken and top with the mozzarella cheese.

5. Return to the oven and bake until the cheese melts, an additional 5 to 7 minutes.

PREPARATION TIME: **10 MINUTES**
COOKING TIME: **20 MINUTES**

Moms' Kitchen Notes: Serve with whole wheat spaghetti and a salad.

	Before	After
Calories	450	390
Fat (g)	23	11
Saturated Fat (g)	8	4.5
Sodium (mg)	1,150	610
Carbohydrate (g)	16	12
Fiber (g)	1	1
Protein (g)	44	33

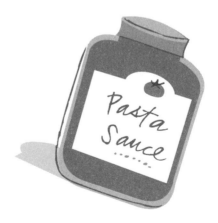

Colorful Cacciatore

MAKES 6 SERVINGS

Chicken cacciatore has plenty of vegetables, but it also has plenty of fat . . . over half a day's worth per serving in fact. The traditional dish calls for a whole chicken (skin and all) cut into pieces and browned in oil. We took the liberty of lightening things up a bit and casually sneaking in one of our favorite, super-nutritious vegetables.

Moms Make It Over By . . .

- Adding bell peppers for vitamins, minerals, phytonutrients, and fiber.
- Using skinless, boneless chicken breast and a moderate amount of healthy olive oil to lower the saturated fat and calories.
- Adding less salt to reduce the sodium.

> ¼ cup all-purpose flour
>
> ½ teaspoon onion powder
>
> ½ teaspoon garlic powder
>
> ½ teaspoon dried oregano
>
> 1½ pounds skinless, boneless chicken breast halves, cut into strips
>
> 1 tablespoon olive oil
>
> One 16-ounce bag frozen mixed bell pepper strips, thawed
>
> One 26-ounce jar pasta sauce
>
> ¼ cup grated Parmesan cheese

1. Combine the flour, onion powder, garlic powder, and oregano in a shallow bowl. Coat the chicken with the flour mixture and shake off excess.

2. Heat the oil in a large nonstick skillet or Dutch oven over medium-high heat. Add the chicken and cook, stirring frequently, until lightly browned, about 3 minutes.

3. Add the bell peppers and cook, stirring frequently, about 3 more minutes.

4. Stir in the pasta sauce and bring to a simmer. Reduce the heat and continue to simmer until the chicken and vegetables are tender, 15 to 20 minutes.

5. Serve in individual bowls and top with Parmesan cheese.

PREPARATION TIME: 10 MINUTES
COOKING TIME: 25 MINUTES

Moms' Kitchen Notes: Serve over couscous or penne pasta.

	Before	After
Calories	650	240
Fat (g)	36	7
Saturated Fat (g)	9	1.5
Sodium (mg)	1,040	500
Carbohydrate (g)	8	17
Fiber (g)	2	4
Protein (g)	65	28

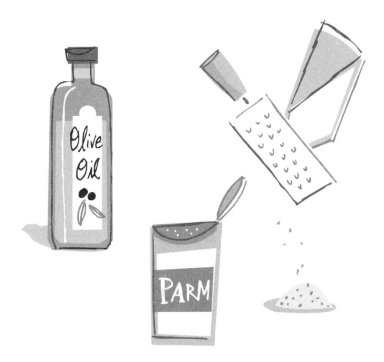

Fit 'n Trim Tetrazzini

MAKES 6 SERVINGS

One day when Janice was leafing through her Nana's old recipe box, she came across a recipe for chicken Tetrazzini. The ingredients made Janice laugh and cringe at the same time because they included such things as cream, butter, Spam, a whole chicken, and a cup of celery. We're sure Nana wouldn't mind, but we couldn't resist adding half a century's worth of changes to her recipe.

Moms Make It Over By . . .

- Adding mushrooms and mixed vegetables for vitamins, minerals, phytonutrients, and fiber.
- Using skinless, boneless chicken breast and lowfat milk to lower the saturated fat.
- Eliminating the Spam and using less added salt to reduce the sodium.

8 ounces dried small-size pasta wheels (about 3 cups)

¼ cup all-purpose flour

1 teaspoon salt

1¼ pounds skinless, boneless chicken breast halves, cut into bite-size pieces

1 tablespoon olive oil

One 8-ounce package presliced mushrooms

2½ cups frozen mixed vegetables, thawed

½ teaspoon garlic powder

½ teaspoon onion powder

½ teaspoon dried Italian seasoning

1 cup 1% lowfat milk

1 tablespoon all-purpose flour

½ cup reduced-fat sour cream

¼ cup grated Parmesan cheese

1. Cook the pasta according to package directions. Drain and return to the pan.

2. While the pasta is cooking, combine the flour and salt in a large bowl. Add the chicken and coat evenly, shaking off excess.

3. Heat the oil in a large nonstick skillet over medium-high heat. Add the chicken and cook, stirring frequently, until lightly browned, about 3 minutes. Add the mushrooms, mixed vegetables, garlic powder, onion powder, and Italian seasoning and cook, stirring frequently, until the mushrooms are tender, 8 to 10 minutes.

4. Meanwhile, combine the milk and flour in a bowl and whisk until well blended. Add to the skillet and bring to a simmer, stirring constantly. Reduce the heat and continue to simmer and stir gently until the sauce thickens, about 2 minutes. Add the sour cream and heat through.

5. Stir the chicken mixture in with the pasta. Serve in individual bowls and top with Parmesan cheese.

PREPARATION TIME: 15 MINUTES
COOKING TIME: 15 MINUTES

	Before	After
Calories	420	380
Fat (g)	25	9
Saturated Fat (g)	11	3.5
Sodium (mg)	1,530	550
Carbohydrate (g)	26	44
Fiber (g)	1	4
Protein (g)	22	31

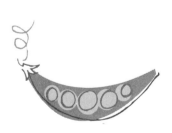

Southwestern Chicken & Rice

MAKES 6 SERVINGS

Every family has a favorite recipe. For Janice's sister, Diane, it's a Southwestern-style chicken and rice dish. When we first tried this recipe, we loved it too, but felt it could use a minor makeover. The original recipe used an entire packet of taco seasoning mix. The mix seemed okay at first glance, but when we read the label and noticed it contained a staggering 3,300 milligrams of sodium along with MSG, we got busy.

Moms Make It Over By ...

- Adding corn for vitamins, minerals, phytonutrients, and fiber.
- Using reduced-fat cheese and reduced-fat sour cream to lower the saturated fat and calories.
- Using instant brown rice for added nutrients and fiber.
- Replacing the taco seasoning mix with a flavorful blend of spices and seasonings to reduce the sodium.

> 1 tablespoon canola oil
>
> 1 pound skinless, boneless chicken breast halves, cut into bite-size pieces
>
> 2 cups frozen corn kernels, thawed
>
> One 15½-ounce can black beans, drained and rinsed
>
> 1½ cups instant brown rice (about 3 cups cooked)
>
> 1½ cups salsa
>
> 1 teaspoon chili powder
>
> 1 teaspoon ground cumin
>
> 1 cup preshredded reduced-fat Cheddar cheese
>
> ½ cup reduced-fat sour cream

1. Heat the oil in a large saucepan or Dutch oven over medium-high heat. Add the chicken and cook, stirring frequently, until lightly browned, about 3 minutes.

2. Stir in the corn, 2 cups water, beans, rice, salsa, chili powder, and cumin and bring to a boil. Reduce the heat and simmer, covered, until the rice is tender, about 15 minutes. Stir in the cheese until melted.

3. Serve in individual bowls and top with sour cream.

PREPARATION TIME: **10 MINUTES**
COOKING TIME: **20 MINUTES**

	Before	After
Calories	540	390
Fat (g)	22	9
Saturated Fat (g)	12	3
Sodium (mg)	1,310	600
Carbohydrate (g)	43	47
Fiber (g)	4	7
Protein (g)	38	31

Moms′ Kitchen Notes: Use pinto beans or black-eyed peas in place of the black beans.

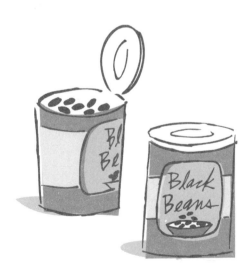

"Mom, the House Smells Great" Roasted Chicken

MAKES 6 SERVINGS

How often have you roasted a chicken only to end up with bland, dried-out cardboard? By no means are we food snobs but we do appreciate good flavor. The secret to our perfect roasted chicken is the aromatic herb, lemon zest, and garlic rub. We also roast the chicken with the skin on to seal in all those great juices.

Moms Make It Over By . . .

- Removing the skin before serving to lower the saturated fat and calories.
- Adding an herb rub to improve the flavor.

> 1½ tablespoons extra virgin olive oil
>
> Zest of 1 lemon
>
> 1 tablespoon finely chopped fresh basil, or 1 teaspoon dried basil
>
> 2 teaspoons finely chopped fresh rosemary, or 1 teaspoon dried rosemary
>
> 1 teaspoon kosher salt
>
> 1 teaspoon bottled crushed garlic, or 1 to 2 garlic cloves, minced
>
> One 4- to 5-pound roasting chicken
>
> Salt and pepper

1. Preheat the oven to 350°F.

2. Combine the oil, lemon zest, basil, rosemary, salt, and garlic in a small bowl and mix well.

3. Place the chicken on a work surface or cutting board. Loosen the skin from the chicken breast and drumsticks by inserting your fingers and gently pushing between the skin and meat.

4. Rub the seasoning mixture under the loosened chicken skin. Sprinkle the chicken with salt and pepper.

5. Place the chicken, breast side up, on a broiler or roasting pan in the center of the oven.

6. Bake until the chicken turns golden brown and an instant-read meat thermometer registers 180°F, about 1 hour and 20 minutes (18 to 20 minutes per pound).

7. Remove and discard the skin. Slice the meat and serve.

PREPARATION TIME: 15 MINUTES

COOKING TIME: 1 HOUR AND 20 MINUTES

	Before	After
Calories	330	190
Fat (g)	19	10
Saturated Fat (g)	5	2
Sodium (mg)	115	380
Carbohydrate (g)	0	1
Fiber (g)	0	0
Protein (g)	38	23

Moms' Kitchen Notes: Serve with Mashed Potatoes with Kale (really!) (page 306).

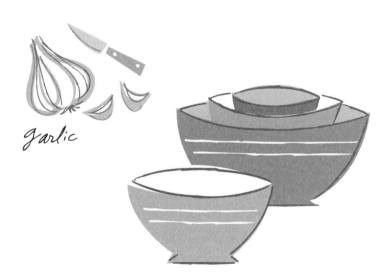

garlic

To Skin or Not to Skin . . . That Is the Question

True or false: It's a good idea to cook chicken with the skin on. The answer, in some cases, is true. Surprised? While cooking chicken with the skin on is often perceived as a nutritional no-no, scientific research (yes, people actually sit around and study this) shows that very little fat from the skin gets absorbed into the chicken meat itself. Instead, the fatty skin acts as a wrap, keeping the meat moist.

Throughout this chapter, we've provided recipes that call for skinless, boneless chicken breast halves, because other ingredients such as tomato sauce and corn flake crumbs are there to coat the meat and keep it juicy. But sometimes it makes great culinary sense to keep the skin on. By no means do we advocate eating chicken skin, because, after all, 80 percent of the fat in chicken is concentrated in the skin. So just remember to remove the skin after the chicken is cooked. Your arteries will surely thank you.

Turkey Meat Loaf Muffins

MAKES 6 SERVINGS

If you've been looking for an alternative to ground beef, chances are you've discovered ground turkey by now. For this recipe, we use it to create a dozen little meat loaf muffins. But there's more to these muffins than the turkey itself with the addition of chopped walnuts, ketchup, honey mustard, and several optional "mix-ins."

Moms Make It Over By . . .

- Switching to lean ground turkey to lower the saturated fat.
- Including walnuts for added nutrients and healthy omega-3 fats.

> 1¼ pounds lean ground turkey
>
> 1 large egg, beaten
>
> 1 cup dried bread crumbs
>
> ½ cup walnuts, finely chopped
>
> ⅓ cup ketchup
>
> 3 tablespoons honey mustard
>
> ¼ teaspoon salt
>
> ½ cup golden raisins, optional
>
> 1 large carrot, shredded, optional (about 1 cup)
>
> 1 cup frozen corn kernels, thawed, optional
>
> ¼ cup preshredded reduced-fat Cheddar cheese

1. Preheat the oven to 375°F.

2. Lightly oil or coat 12 muffin cups with nonstick cooking spray and set aside.

3. Combine the turkey, egg, bread crumbs, walnuts, ketchup, honey mustard, salt, and your choice of raisins, carrot, or corn as desired in a large bowl and mix well.

4. Divide the turkey mixture evenly among the muffin cups and top each with a teaspoon of the cheese. Bake until an instant-read thermometer registers 165°F, about 30 minutes.

PREPARATION TIME: 15 MINUTES
COOKING TIME: 30 MINUTES

	Before	After
Calories	330	360
Fat (g)	21	18
Saturated Fat (g)	8	3.5
Sodium (mg)	620	560
Carbohydrate (g)	16	27
Fiber (g)	2	2
Protein (g)	20	23

Jolly Green Bean & Chicken Casserole

MAKES 6 SERVINGS

Green bean casserole is one of those all-American favorites that hasn't really changed much since the 1940s. Traditionally made with canned green beans, cream of mushroom soup, and fried onions on top, we couldn't wait to get our kitchen mitts on this one. You'll love our new-and-improved classic (which, by the way, we've turned into an entrée).

Moms Make It Over By . . .

🍓 Including chicken for added protein.

🍓 Using almonds for added nutrients and heart-healthy monounsaturated fats.

2 cups corn flakes

¼ cup sliced almonds

1 tablespoon olive oil

1½ pounds skinless, boneless chicken breast halves, cut into bite-size pieces

One 10-ounce package presliced mushrooms

1 teaspoon bottled crushed garlic, or 1 to 2 garlic cloves, minced

1 teaspoon onion powder

1 teaspoon dried tarragon

1 teaspoon salt

2 cups 1% lowfat milk

⅓ cup all-purpose flour

Two 9-ounce packages frozen French cut green beans, thawed and drained

¼ cup grated Parmesan cheese

1. Combine the corn flakes and almonds in a food processor and pulse a few turns until coarsely crushed. Set aside.

2. Preheat the oven to 425°F.

3. Heat the oil in a large nonstick skillet over medium-high heat. Add the chicken and cook until lightly browned, stirring frequently, about 3 minutes. Add the mushrooms, garlic, onion powder, tarragon, and salt and cook until the mushrooms are tender and the chicken is no longer pink, about 6 minutes.

4. While the chicken is cooking, whisk together the milk and flour in a medium bowl until well blended. When the chicken and mushrooms are done, add the milk mixture (rewhisk if necessary) to the skillet and bring to a simmer, stirring constantly. Reduce the heat and continue to simmer and stir gently until the liquid thickens, about 2 minutes.

5. To assemble, place the green beans in a 9 x 13-inch baking pan. Arrange the chicken mixture evenly over the top. Sprinkle with the Parmesan cheese and the corn flake mixture and bake until heated through, about 15 minutes.

PREPARATION TIME: 25 MINUTES
COOKING TIME: 15 MINUTES

Moms' Kitchen Notes: Serve over rice.

	Before	After
Calories	180	320
Fat (g)	11	10
Saturated Fat (g)	3	2.5
Sodium (mg)	820	620
Carbohydrate (g)	16	26
Fiber (g)	3	3
Protein (g)	4	32

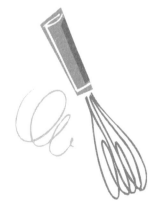

CHAPTER 13

Simply Sensible Side Dishes

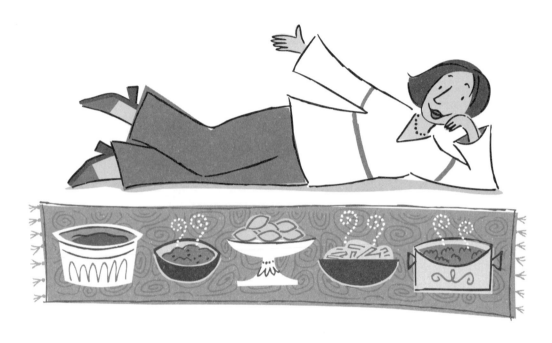

Scalloped Spuds with Broccoli • Sweet Potato Fries • Mashed Potatoes with Kale (really!) • Honey Wheat Popovers • Sweet & Nutty Couscous • Olive Oil's Orzo • Bulgur & Carrot Pilaf • Maple-Glazed Carrots • Cheesy Cauliflower • Garlicky Sautéed Spinach • Finally Edible Brussels Sprouts • Sunny Broccoli Stew

S ide dishes can make a nutritional fashion statement. But in many of today's households, cooked vegetables and potatoes, salads, breads, and other supper side dishes have been nixed from the family dinner table. The reason: prep time and clean up. While we can't blame parents for doing whatever it takes to streamline the evening meal, side dishes offer an amazing opportunity to weave in super nutrition. To save the side dish from extinction, consider a simple side of colorful berries or sweet melon, or try our Maple-Glazed Carrots (page 313), Garlicky Sautéed Spinach (page 316), or oven-baked Sweet Potato Fries (page 304). If you've made a commitment to a family meal makeover, a nutrient-packed side dish can often come to the rescue. Remember that minimum of 5 servings of fruits and vegetables we're all supposed to be eating each day? Well, reaching that goal gets a whole lot easier when they're served on the side.

It's easy to accessorize your meals with healthy side dishes, especially when you're armed with fast and easy recipes. Many of our creations utilize frozen vegetables or fresh prepared produce such as the prewashed baby spinach and scalloped potatoes now available in most supermarkets. There's also the supermarket salad bar for busy moms in a bind. There, you'll find prechopped fruits and veggies that require minimal prep time. A word of caution, however. Salad bar fare can be high in saturated fat and sodium, especially if you gravitate to the creamy potato and macaroni salads.

In this chapter, we present a side dish for every occasion . . . from quick weeknight meals to backyard barbeques. Scalloped potatoes, for example, that time-honored side dish traditionally made with lots of heavy cream, receives a much-needed renovation with a simple combination of lighter ingredients that offer the same rich appeal. Even coleslaw gets an overhaul. Instead of grabbing a pint from the deli counter, we make it from scratch using broccoli coleslaw, a nutritional superstar in the supermarket produce aisle.

We make vegetables fun and delicious without smothering them in rich buttery cream sauces. We even have a few tricks up our sleeve for getting children (and adults) to eat and love Brussels sprouts, kale, and cauliflower! Now that's progress. So if you're looking for a way to kick up your meals a few nutritional notches, stick with side dishes . . . just choose them wisely.

Scalloped Spuds with Broccoli

MAKES 6 SERVINGS

When thin slices of potato are layered in a casserole dish and then covered with heavy cream and butter, what you get is 20 grams of fat in a serving and a dish known as scalloped potatoes. It's a classic side dish screaming for a makeover. Keeping the creaminess in, while evicting the butter and cream, was a challenge—you should have heard the Meal Makeover Moms bickering over this one! But we compromised and in the end, even tossed in some broccoli to boot.

Moms Make It Over By ...

- Adding broccoli for vitamins, minerals, phytonutrients, and fiber.
- Using lowfat milk and reduced-fat cheese to lower the saturated fat and calories.

> ¼ cup all-purpose flour
>
> 1 teaspoon salt
>
> ½ teaspoon garlic powder
>
> ⅛ teaspoon ground nutmeg
>
> Pinch of pepper
>
> One 24-ounce bag refrigerated scallop cut potatoes
>
> One 14- or 16-ounce bag frozen broccoli florets, thawed
>
> 1 cup preshredded reduced-fat Cheddar cheese
>
> 1½ cups 1% lowfat milk
>
> ¼ cup grated Parmesan cheese
>
> 2 tablespoons dried seasoned bread crumbs

1. Preheat the oven to 425°F.

2. Lightly oil or coat a 9 x 13-inch baking pan with nonstick cooking spray and set aside.

3. Whisk together the flour, salt, garlic powder, nutmeg, and pepper in a large bowl until well blended.

4. Add the potatoes, broccoli, and Cheddar cheese and toss to coat.

5. Arrange the potato mixture in the baking pan and pour the milk over the top. Sprinkle evenly with Parmesan cheese and bread crumbs.

6. Bake uncovered until the potatoes are tender and golden brown, about 30 minutes. Let stand 5 minutes before serving.

PREPARATION TIME: **10 MINUTES**
COOKING TIME: **30 MINUTES**

Moms' Kitchen Notes: Serve with grilled steak or seafood.

	Before	After
Calories	390	210
Fat (g)	21	5
Saturated Fat (g)	11	3
Sodium (mg)	1,180	660
Carbohydrate (g)	35	33
Fiber (g)	3	5
Protein (g)	21	14

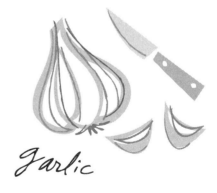

garlic

Sweet Potato Fries

MAKES 4 SERVINGS

At mealtime, children are more likely to eat French fries than any other vegetable . . . a fact that motivated us to create a more nourishing alternative to all those frozen French fries, potato puffs, and Tater Tots from the supermarket freezer section. Our homemade Sweet Potato Fries are easy to make, kids gobble them up, and they're off the charts when it comes to things like beta-carotene. If you have a rule in your house that the kids can't eat with their fingers, break it for these delicious fries.

Moms Make It Over By . . .

- Using sweet potatoes for added vitamins, minerals, phytonutrients, and fiber.
- Cooking in a moderate amount of healthy olive oil to eliminate the saturated fat and eliminate the trans fats.

2 large sweet potatoes, peeled

1 to 2 tablespoons olive oil or canola oil

½ teaspoon salt

½ teaspoon ground cinnamon

¼ teaspoon ground ginger

	Before	After
Calories	170	120
Fat (g)	8	3.5
Saturated Fat (g)	1.5	0
Sodium (mg)	440	300
Carbohydrate (g)	21	22
Fiber (g)	2	3
Protein (g)	1	2

1. Preheat the oven to 425°F.

2. Cut the sweet potatoes in half lengthwise, then cut each half into 6 wedges.

3. Combine the oil, salt, cinnamon, and ginger in a large shallow bowl and mix well. Add the sweet potatoes and toss to coat evenly with the oil mixture.

4. Place the wedges in a single layer on a baking sheet. Bake for 25 minutes or until tender.

PREPARATION TIME: **10 MINUTES**
COOKING TIME: **25 MINUTES**

Moms' Kitchen Notes: Dip in pure maple syrup for some extra sweetness.

Pump Up the Produce: Supersize Your Portions

Americans have grown accustomed to supersized portions. A medium bag of movie theater popcorn back in the 1950s contained 3 cups . . . now it overflows with 16. A fast food soft drink 50 years ago was 8 ounces but today it can be four times that size. You get the picture. Well, now we're here to tell you that supersizing is a great idea . . . as long as you reserve it for produce.

- Pasta with tomato sauce (1 serving) + 1 cup broccoli (2 servings) = 3 produce servings
- Baked apple (1 serving) + ¼ cup raisins (1 serving) = 2 produce servings
- 1 small green salad (1 serving) + ½ cup shredded carrots (1 serving) + ½ cup grape tomatoes (1 serving) = 3 produce servings
- 1 fruit juice smoothie with 1 medium banana (2 servings) + ½ cup frozen strawberries (1 serving) = 3 produce servings

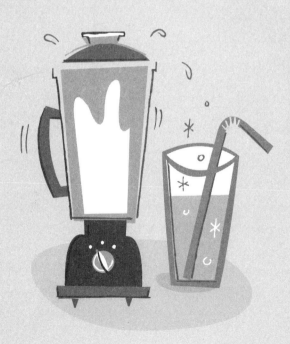

Mashed Potatoes with Kale (really!)

MAKES 6 SERVINGS

If there is one vegetable we should all be eating more of, it is kale—rich in carotenoids, vitamin C, and vitamin K . . . a nutrient good for bone health. That's the upside. The downside to kale, however, is the fact that it takes a bit of time to wash, clean, chop, and cook. So for this recipe we took a shortcut by using frozen kale. Mixing it into mashed potatoes may seem bizarre but the result is surprisingly delicious. You may need to do some clever marketing to get your family to try this dish but once they take that very first bite, they'll become kale lovers for life. Really!

Moms Make It Over By . . .

🥕 Adding kale for vitamins, minerals, phytonutrients, and fiber.

🥕 Using chicken broth instead of cream to lower the saturated fat and calories.

One 10-ounce box frozen chopped kale

3 pounds potatoes, peeled and cut into ½-inch cubes (6 to 7 cups)

⅔ cup all-natural chicken broth

¼ cup grated Parmesan cheese

1 tablespoon butter

½ teaspoon salt

¼ teaspoon garlic powder

Pepper

1. Cook the kale according to package directions. Drain in a colander and squeeze out any excess liquid.

2. While the kale is cooking, place the potatoes in a large saucepan. Add enough water to cover. Cover and bring to a boil. Reduce the heat and cook, covered, at a low boil until tender, about 10 minutes.

3. When the potatoes are done, drain and return to the pan. Add the broth, Parmesan cheese, butter, salt, and garlic powder and, using a potato masher, mash until smooth.

4. Add the kale and stir to combine. Season with pepper to taste.

PREPARATION TIME: 15 MINUTES
COOKING TIME: 20 MINUTES

Moms' Kitchen Notes: Lowfat milk can be substituted for the chicken broth.

	Before	After
Calories	250	210
Fat (g)	15	1.5
Saturated Fat (g)	9	0.5
Sodium (mg)	500	340
Carbohydrate (g)	28	44
Fiber (g)	2	4
Protein (g)	4	8

Kick Up the K

What do kale, spinach, collard greens, romaine lettuce, Brussels sprouts, and broccoli have in common? Besides the fact that they're all green, they are some of the best food sources of vitamin K in the supermarket. Vitamin K isn't exactly coffee klatch conversation, but maybe it should be. It turns out that this often-forgotten vitamin seems to protect against hip fractures.

Americans don't get enough vitamin K . . . no big surprise given that most people don't eat their greens every day. Our advice: Eat one vitamin K–rich food on most days to protect your bones.

Honey Wheat Popovers

MAKES 5 SERVINGS (2 POPOVERS EACH)

There's something magical about popovers. They start out as batter and quickly puff up into whimsical little breads. Popovers are ideal accompaniments to soups and stews . . . coming in handy when it's time to lap up those last tenacious drops. The original popover recipe, made with white flour, eggs, and milk, was far from a diet disaster, but we figured a little dollop of fiber couldn't hurt.

Moms Make It Over By . . .

🦋 Using whole wheat flour for added nutrients and fiber.

> 1 tablespoon butter, melted
> 2/3 cup all-purpose flour
> 1/3 cup whole wheat flour
> 1/4 teaspoon salt
> 1 cup 1% lowfat milk
> 2 large eggs, beaten
> 1 tablespoon honey

1. Preheat the oven to 375°F.

2. Brush the insides of 10 muffin cups very well with the melted butter. Set aside.

3. Whisk together the all-purpose flour, whole wheat flour, and salt in a medium bowl.

4. Whisk together the milk, eggs, and honey in a medium bowl. Add the flour mixture and whisk until smooth.

5. Pour the batter into the muffin cups, filling each about half full.

6. Bake for 30 minutes or until puffed and golden. Serve immediately.

PREPARATION TIME: **10 MINUTES**
COOKING TIME: **30 MINUTES**

	Before	After
Calories	180	170
Fat (g)	7	5
Saturated Fat (g)	3.5	2.5
Sodium (mg)	290	190
Carbohydrate (g)	22	24
Fiber (g)	<1	1
Protein (g)	7	7

Sweet & Nutty Couscous

MAKES 4 TO 5 SERVINGS

Nothing could be easier than cooking up a box of plain old couscous but then again, it's nice to go "out of the box" once in a while. We've taken couscous and kicked it up a flavor notch. And by using whole wheat couscous, we've kicked up the fiber as well.

Moms Make It Over By . . .

- Adding peas for vitamins, minerals, phytonutrients, and fiber.
- Using whole wheat couscous for added nutrients and fiber.
- Including pecans for added nutrients and heart-healthy monounsaturated fats.

1 cup apple juice

¼ teaspoon salt

⅛ teaspoon ground cinnamon

1 cup frozen peas, thawed

¾ cup whole wheat couscous

¼ cup golden raisins

⅓ cup pecans, toasted and coarsely chopped

1. Combine the apple juice, ½ cup water, salt, and cinnamon in a medium saucepan and bring to a boil. Remove from the heat and stir in the peas, couscous, and raisins. Cover and let stand 5 to 10 minutes.

2. Fluff the couscous with a fork, stir in the pecans, and serve.

PREPARATION TIME: 15 MINUTES

	Before	After
Calories	230	270
Fat (g)	2	7
Saturated Fat (g)	0	0.5
Sodium (mg)	5	160
Carbohydrate (g)	46	49
Fiber (g)	2	8
Protein (g)	8	8

Olive Oil's Orzo

MAKES 6 SERVINGS

Bored with buttered noodles? If you are, then use olive oil instead. But don't stop there. Do what we did and take the best of the Mediterranean—pasta, greens, nuts, and olives—and blend it all together for one amazingly flavorful side dish. Between all the healthy fats in the oil and the antioxidants in the greens, you'll be a giant step closer to your family meal makeover.

Moms Make It Over By . . .

- Adding spinach for vitamins, minerals, phytonutrients, and fiber.
- Using a moderate amount of healthy olive oil to lower the saturated fat.

> **10 ounces dried orzo (about 1½ cups)**
>
> **One 6-ounce bag prewashed baby spinach (about 4 packed cups)**
>
> **⅓ cup pine nuts, lightly toasted**
>
> **¼ cup pitted kalamata olives, chopped**
>
> **¼ cup grated Parmesan cheese**
>
> **3 tablespoons olive oil**
>
> **3 tablespoons balsamic vinegar**
>
> **½ teaspoon kosher salt**
>
> **¼ teaspoon garlic powder**

1. Cook the pasta according to package directions. Drain and immediately return to the hot pan.

2. Add the spinach and toss until the leaves wilt.

3. Add the pine nuts, olives, Parmesan cheese, oil, vinegar, salt, and garlic powder and mix until well combined.

4. Serve hot or refrigerate for several hours and serve chilled.

PREPARATION TIME: 10 MINUTES

COOKING TIME: 10 MINUTES

Moms' Kitchen Notes: If your children are adventurous eaters, add ¼ cup chopped sun-dried tomatoes, fresh chopped basil, or diced yellow bell pepper.

	Before	After
Calories	330	320
Fat (g)	15	14
Saturated Fat (g)	9	2.5
Sodium (mg)	480	290
Carbohydrate (g)	39	39
Fiber (g)	2	2
Protein (g)	8	10

Bulgur & Carrot Pilaf

MAKES 5 SERVINGS

Are you stuck in a rice rut? While rice is easy to make (hey, you can even boil it in a bag!) and children usually like it, eating it night after night can get a bit monotonous. To shake things up a bit at your table, try bulgur . . . a whole grain with a mild, nutty flavor. Bulgur is made from fiber-rich whole wheat kernels that have been steamed, dried, and crushed.

Moms Make It Over By . . .

- Adding carrot for vitamins, minerals, phytonutrients, and fiber.
- Switching to bulgur for added nutrients and fiber.

> 1 tablespoon olive oil
>
> 1 tablespoon butter
>
> 2 ounces fine egg noodles (about 1 cup)
>
> 1 large carrot, shredded (about 1 cup)
>
> 1 cup bulgur
>
> 2 cups all-natural chicken broth or vegetable broth

1. Heat the oil and butter in a medium saucepan over medium-high heat. When the butter melts, add the noodles and cook, stirring constantly, until lightly browned, about 2 minutes.

2. Stir in the carrot and bulgur. Add the broth and bring to a boil. Reduce the heat and simmer, covered, stirring frequently, until the liquid is absorbed, about 20 minutes.

PREPARATION TIME: 5 MINUTES
COOKING TIME: 25 MINUTES

	Before	After
Calories	160	200
Fat (g)	0	6
Saturated Fat (g)	0	2
Sodium (mg)	0	270
Carbohydrate (g)	35	32
Fiber (g)	0	7
Protein (g)	3	6

Moms' Kitchen Notes: Serve with Grilled Salmon with Ginger Honey Glaze (page 257).

Maple-Glazed Carrots

MAKES 4 SERVINGS

"**O**h, Mom. Not steamed carrots *again!*" Sound familiar? Steamed veggies can get kind of old after a while. That's why some moms smother them with butter and salt so their kids will eat them. For a healthier and more flavorful solution to your carrot woes, dress them up with maple syrup and apple juice instead. A minor flavor makeover turns nutrient-rich carrots into a must-have side dish that no one will complain about.

Moms Make It Over By ...

❤ Using less butter to lower the saturated fat.

> One 10-ounce bag carrot sticks, or 3 large carrots, quartered
>   lengthwise and cut into 4-inch sticks
>
> ⅔ cup apple juice
>
> ¼ teaspoon salt
>
> 1 to 2 tablespoons pure maple syrup
>
> 1 teaspoon butter

1. Add the carrots, apple juice, and salt to a large nonstick skillet and cook over medium-high heat, stirring frequently, until the carrots are tender, about 10 minutes. Add extra juice or water if all the liquid evaporates.

2. Stir in the maple syrup and butter and continue to cook until the butter melts, about 1 minute.

PREPARATION TIME: 5 MINUTES
COOKING TIME: 10 MINUTES

	Before	After
Calories	140	70
Fat (g)	11	1
Saturated Fat (g)	7	0.5
Sodium (mg)	350	180
Carbohydrate (g)	8	15
Fiber (g)	2	2
Protein (g)	1	1

Moms' Kitchen Notes: Serve with Walnut-Crusted Salmon (page 258).

Cheesy Cauliflower

MAKES 6 SERVINGS

Back when Janice was in college, her favorite meal consisted of platefuls of fried cauliflower dipped in ketchup. Well, even though the fried stuff had more fat than her shiny new college calculator could tally, she had all the right intentions: trying to eat her vegetables just like Mom told her to. Today, cauliflower is still a biggie with Janice, but instead of a deep-fat fryer, she uses this sumptuous cheese sauce.

Moms Make It Over By . . .

- ♨ Steaming versus frying to lower the total fat and calories.
- ♨ Creating a cheese sauce with lowfat milk and reduced-fat cheese to add bone-building calcium.

> One 16- or 20-ounce bag frozen cauliflower florets, or 1 small head
>   cauliflower, broken into florets
>
> 3/4 cup 1% lowfat milk
>
> 1 tablespoon all-purpose flour
>
> 1/2 teaspoon Dijon mustard
>
> 1/8 teaspoon garlic powder
>
> 3/4 cup preshredded reduced-fat Cheddar cheese
>
> 2 tablespoons grated Parmesan cheese
>
> 2 tablespoons dried plain or seasoned bread crumbs

1. Cook the cauliflower according to package directions or steam fresh cauliflower until tender, 8 to 10 minutes. Set aside.

2. While the cauliflower is cooking, whisk together the milk, flour, mustard, and garlic powder in a small saucepan until well blended. Place over medium-high heat and bring to a simmer, stirring constantly. Reduce the heat and continue to simmer and stir gently until the mixture thickens slightly, about 2 minutes.

3. Stir in the Cheddar cheese and Parmesan cheese until melted.

4. Preheat the broiler on high.

5. Arrange the cauliflower in a baking pan and pour the cheese sauce evenly over the top. Sprinkle with the bread crumbs and broil until the bread crumbs turn golden brown, about 2 minutes.

PREPARATION TIME: 5 MINUTES
COOKING TIME: 15 MINUTES

Moms' Kitchen Notes: Serve with Turkey Meat Loaf Muffins (page 297).

	Before	After
Calories	260	140
Fat (g)	20	2.5
Saturated Fat (g)	4.5	1
Sodium (mg)	240	80
Carbohydrate (g)	17	21
Fiber (g)	2	2
Protein (g)	6	9

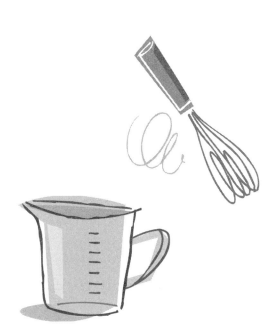

Garlicky Sautéed Spinach

MAKES 4 SERVINGS

If there's one scary food memory from our childhoods it's got to be creamed spinach. If you were traumatized by creamed spinach like we were, it's time to move on and get some closure with our Garlicky Sautéed Spinach. This recipe is so simple that the natural flavors of the spinach are allowed to shine through. No creamy green stuff for our kids!

Moms Make It Over By . . .

🍓 Cooking in a moderate amount of healthy olive oil to lower the saturated fat and calories.

> 1 tablespoon extra virgin olive oil
> ½ teaspoon bottled crushed garlic, or 1 garlic clove, minced
> One 9-ounce bag prewashed baby spinach (about 6 packed cups)
> Pinch of kosher salt

1. Heat the oil in a large saucepan over medium-low heat.

2. Add the garlic and cook until golden, about 1 minute. Add the spinach, raise the heat to medium, and cook, stirring frequently, until the spinach wilts and is fully cooked, 4 to 5 minutes.

3. Season with salt to taste.

PREPARATION TIME: 5 MINUTES
COOKING TIME: 5 MINUTES

	Before	After
Calories	120	45
Fat (g)	11	3.5
Saturated Fat (g)	7	0
Sodium (mg)	310	105
Carbohydrate (g)	4	3
Fiber (g)	2	2
Protein (g)	3	2

Moms' Kitchen Notes: If you can't find a bag of the prewashed baby spinach, buy the regular bagged stuff instead . . . just be sure to trim off the woody stems.

Finally Edible Brussels Sprouts

MAKES 4 SERVINGS

Okay. How many children in this country, or for that matter, on the planet, *like* Brussels sprouts? We know of two: Liz's boys. Her recipe, which she got from a family friend, turns Brussels sprouts into an irresistible side dish. The original recipe, admittedly, had ½ stick of butter, but slimming it down without losing the flavor was actually quite easy. Oh, and with 6 grams of fiber and a healthy burst of vitamin K, it's worth the effort to try this dish at least once.

Moms Make It Over By . . .

- Using less butter and a small amount of healthy olive oil to lower the saturated fat and calories.

> 1½ pounds Brussels sprouts
>
> 1 tablespoon olive oil
>
> ½ tablespoon butter
>
> 1 teaspoon bottled crushed garlic, or 1 to 2 garlic cloves, minced
>
> ¼ cup pine nuts
>
> 2 tablespoons grated Parmesan cheese
>
> ¼ teaspoon kosher salt

1. Trim off the stem ends of the Brussels sprouts using a sharp knife. Peel off the loose leaves from around the stems and slice each sprout in half lengthwise. Wash and drain.

2. Steam the Brussels sprouts until very soft, 20 to 25 minutes.

3. A few minutes before the sprouts are done, heat the oil and butter in a large nonstick skillet over medium-low heat. Add the garlic and pine nuts and cook until the garlic turns golden brown, about 2 minutes.

4. Transfer the Brussels sprouts to the skillet. Toss with the pine nut mixture and sprinkle with the Parmesan cheese and salt. Serve hot.

	Before	After
Calories	240	170
Fat (g)	18	10
Saturated Fat (g)	9	2.5
Sodium (mg)	540	190
Carbohydrate (g)	15	15
Fiber (g)	6	6
Protein (g)	9	8

PREPARATION TIME: 10 MINUTES
COOKING TIME: 25 MINUTES

Simply Delicious Broccoli

Spinach isn't the only vegetable that tastes better with the addition of extra virgin olive oil and kosher salt. If your children have a green vegetable "phobia," here's a simple recipe that is sure to cure them.

1 head broccoli, cut into florets (5 to 6 cups)

1 to 2 tablespoons extra virgin olive oil

A few pinches of kosher salt

Steam the broccoli until tender, 5 to 7 minutes. Transfer to a large serving bowl and drizzle with the oil. Sprinkle with salt and toss to coat evenly.

Sunny Broccoli Slaw

MAKES 6 SERVINGS

Coleslaw is a no-brainer. All you have to do is stroll by the supermarket deli counter and ask for it. Well, unfortunately that no-brainer is usually chock full of fat and calories. No need to pout. Instead of deli slaw, we created a new kind of side dish using broccoli coleslaw. You can find this nutritional superstar in the refrigerated section of the produce aisle next to the bags of prewashed salad greens and baby carrots. It's convenience at its best.

Moms Make It Over By . . .

- Using broccoli coleslaw, raisins, and sunflower seeds for vitamins, minerals, phytonutrients, and fiber.
- Using light canola mayonnaise to lower the calories.

> **One 16-ounce bag broccoli coleslaw**
> **½ cup golden raisins**
> **½ cup roasted, shelled sunflower seeds**
> **½ cup light canola mayonnaise**
> **3 tablespoons red wine vinegar**
> **2 tablespoons sugar**
> **½ teaspoon salt**

1. Combine the broccoli coleslaw, raisins, sunflower seeds, mayonnaise, vinegar, sugar, and salt in a large bowl and mix until well blended.

2. Serve right away or refrigerate and serve chilled.

PREPARATION TIME: 10 MINUTES

	Before	After
Calories	250	190
Fat (g)	22	10
Saturated Fat (g)	3	0.5
Sodium (mg)	570	300
Carbohydrate (g)	10	22
Fiber (g)	3	4
Protein (g)	1	5

Moms' Kitchen Notes: Serve with Cheesy Black Bean Burgers (page 222).

CHAPTER 14

Deliciously Smart Desserts

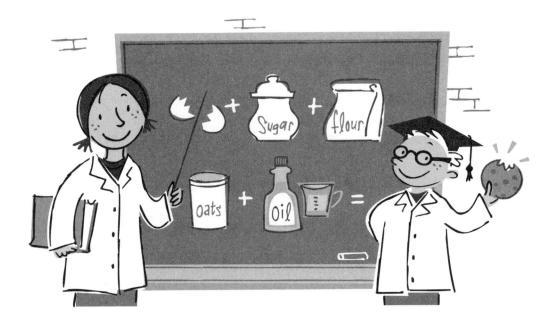

Chocolate Pudding with Toppers • Our Favorite Chocolate Cookie • Oatmeal Mini Chocolate Chip Cookies • Crispy Cereal Treats • Blueberry Snack Cake • Brownie Mix Makeover • I-Can't-Believe-It's Bread Pudding • Chocolate-Dipped Strawberries • Apple & Pear Crisp • Carrot Cake with Lemony Glaze • Banana Chocolate Chip Muffins • Better-Than-Store-Bought "Jell-O"

Ah, dessert. As children, we remember coming home to the aroma of freshly baked cookies and the pleasure of taking those first gooey bites. Today, we enjoy our own children's company at the kitchen counter, though the room inevitably gets coated with a thin dusting of flour and doughy fingerprints land all over the walls. For some moms, however, desserts—instead of bringing on the nostalgia—bring on the guilt . . . especially when they're loaded with butter, sugar, and cream.

Our dessert makeovers illustrate how sweet treats don't have to be forbidden fruit but rather a way to incorporate feel-good flavors as well as super nutrition into your family's diet. Indeed, all of our awesome desserts go light on the saturated fat from butter and cream, but we more than make up for it. Our recipes are bursting with fiber as well as healthy omega-3 fats and monounsaturated fats from the canola oil and olive oil that we often use in lieu of butter. They're also brimming with other health-enhancing nutrients found in whole wheat flour, nuts, wheat germ, fruits, and vegetables (yes, sometimes we even toss in a vegetable). Don't get the wrong idea here. These are not sugar-free, cardboard-tasting desserts. They are sweet (yes, we use sugar) and delicious.

The treats in this chapter help to bring the art of baking back to the family kitchen. Take our Oatmeal Mini Chocolate Chip Cookies (page 326), for example, a lighter, nutritionally revved-up version of the time-honored Toll House cookie. Instead of the requisite two sticks of butter, we use $1/2$ cup of canola oil. It's a surprising switch but it works wonders in these impossible-to-resist cookies. Our Brownie Mix Makeover (page 332) is also a surprise, with our "healthy" brownie mix (can you believe we actually found one without trans fats?), a mashed banana mixed right in, and some wheat germ for heart-healthy vitamin E. We've served these brownies to dozens of kids and they're always a huge hit. These are not desserts to die for but rather to live a healthier life by.

Chocolate Pudding with Toppers

MAKES SIX ½-CUP SERVINGS

One of the easiest ways to make chocolate pudding for the kids is to grab a 50-cent box of instant pudding mix. You can't beat the convenience, but with it can come artificial flavors and colors, including red 40, yellow 5, and blue 1. What's up with that? For an all-natural alternative, take a few extra minutes and make our chocolate pudding from scratch. Topped with your choice of add-ins, such as nuts, raisins, or sliced fresh fruit, it's a tempting ending to any meal.

Moms Make It Over By . . .

- Using 1% lowfat milk to lower the saturated fat.
- Making it from scratch to eliminate the artificial flavors and colors.

½ cup sugar

⅓ cup unsweetened cocoa powder

3 tablespoons cornstarch

⅛ teaspoon salt

2½ cups 1% lowfat milk

½ cup lowfat vanilla yogurt

1 teaspoon vanilla extract

Toppings (optional)

Graham crackers, crushed

Chopped nuts

Granola

Fresh fruit, such as sliced bananas or berries

Whipped light cream

1. Whisk together the sugar, cocoa, cornstarch, and salt in a medium saucepan.

2. Gradually whisk in the milk until well blended. Place over medium-high heat and bring to a simmer, stirring constantly. Reduce the heat and continue to simmer, stirring gently, until the mixture thickens slightly, about 2 minutes.

3. Remove from the heat and stir in the yogurt and vanilla.

4. Spoon the mixture into 6 individual serving bowls. Cover with plastic wrap or wax paper (this will prevent a film from forming) and chill for at least 1 hour.

5. Sprinkle with toppings as desired and serve.

PREPARATION TIME: 5 MINUTES
COOKING TIME: 10 MINUTES

Moms' Kitchen Notes: Set up small bowls with several toppings and let the kids help by topping their own pudding.

	Before	After
Calories	170	160
Fat (g)	4.5	1.5
Saturated Fat (g)	2.5	1
Sodium (mg)	450	115
Carbohydrate (g)	30	31
Fiber (g)	1	1
Protein (g)	5	5

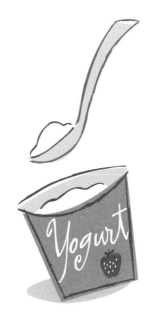

Our Favorite Chocolate Cookie

MAKES FOUR DOZEN 2-INCH COOKIES (2 PER SERVING)

Every Christmas, Janice joins her neighborhood cookie swap, and every year she makes the same thing: her favorite chocolate crinkle cookie. The ingredients are nothing out of the ordinary—butter, cocoa, and sugar—but her cookies are always a huge hit. When we set out to create the dessert recipes for this chapter, those infamous crinkle cookies were one of the first on our list to make over. Guess what Janice is swapping at Christmas this year? Good nutrition.

Moms Make It Over By . . .

- Using whole wheat flour for added nutrients and fiber.
- Using canola oil to lower the saturated fat and increase the healthy omega-3 fats.
- Including pecans for added nutrients and heart-healthy monounsaturated fats.

    1 cup all-purpose flour

    3/4 cup whole wheat flour

    1/2 cup unsweetened cocoa powder

    1 teaspoon baking soda

    1/2 teaspoon salt

    1 cup packed brown sugar

    2/3 cup canola oil

    2 large eggs

    1 teaspoon vanilla extract

    1 cup pecans, very finely chopped

    3 tablespoons granulated sugar

1. Preheat the oven to 350°F.

2. Lightly oil or coat two large baking sheets with nonstick cooking spray and set aside.

3. Whisk together the flour, whole wheat flour, cocoa, baking soda, and salt in a large bowl and set aside.

4. Combine the brown sugar and oil in a large bowl and beat on medium speed until moistened and combined, 1 to 2 minutes. Add the eggs and vanilla and continue to beat until smooth. Scrape down the sides of the bowl if necessary.

5. At low speed, gradually beat in the flour mixture until just combined. Stir in the pecans.

6. Pour the granulated sugar onto a plate. Roll the dough into 1-inch balls and coat evenly with the sugar. Place the cookies on the prepared baking sheets, leaving space in between. Flatten the cookies slightly with the palm of your hand.

7. Bake for 8 to 10 minutes. Transfer the cookies to a wire rack and cool for 5 minutes before serving. Repeat with the remaining dough.

PREPARATION TIME: 20 MINUTES
COOKING TIME: 30 MINUTES

	Before	After
Calories	200	170
Fat (g)	9	11
Saturated Fat (g)	5	1
Sodium (mg)	170	110
Carbohydrate (g)	30	19
Fiber (g)	1	2
Protein (g)	3	2

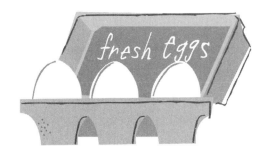

Oatmeal Mini Chocolate Chip Cookies

MAKES THREE DOZEN 2-INCH COOKIES (1 PER SERVING)

Janice grew up making Toll House cookies with her mom but hesitates to do the same with her own children today given the 2 sticks of butter and 2 cups of chocolate chips in the original recipe. The solution to her baking dilemma is our revamped, equally delicious recipe, made with hearty oats and ½ cup of canola oil.

Moms Make It Over By ...

- Using canola oil to lower the saturated fat and increase the omega-3 healthy fats.
- Including walnuts for added nutrients and healthy omega-3 fats.

> **3 cups quick-cooking oats**
> **1 cup all-purpose flour**
> **1 teaspoon baking soda**
> **½ teaspoon salt**
> **½ teaspoon ground cinnamon**
> **1¼ cups packed brown sugar**
> **½ cup canola oil or olive oil**
> **2 large eggs**
> **1 teaspoon vanilla extract**
> **¾ cup walnuts, very finely chopped**
> **½ cup mini chocolate chips**

1. Preheat the oven to 375°F.
2. Lightly oil or coat two large baking sheets with nonstick cooking spray and set aside.
3. Whisk together the oats, flour, baking soda, salt, and cinnamon in a large bowl.
4. Combine the sugar and oil in a large bowl and beat on medium speed until well blended, 1 minute. Add the eggs and vanilla and continue to beat until smooth. Scrape down the sides of the bowl if necessary.
5. At low speed, gradually beat in the oat mixture until just combined. Beat or stir in the walnuts and chocolate chips.

6. Drop by rounded tablespoon onto the prepared baking sheets, leaving space in between. Bake for 10 to 12 minutes, until golden brown. Transfer the cookies to a wire rack and cool for 5 minutes before serving. Repeat with the remaining batter.

PREPARATION TIME: 20 MINUTES
COOKING TIME: 35 MINUTES

	Before	After
Calories	140	120
Fat (g)	8	6
Saturated Fat (g)	4	1
Sodium (mg)	120	75
Carbohydrate (g)	16	15
Fiber (g)	<1	1
Protein (g)	2	2

Moms' Kitchen Notes: For a change of pace, add raisins.

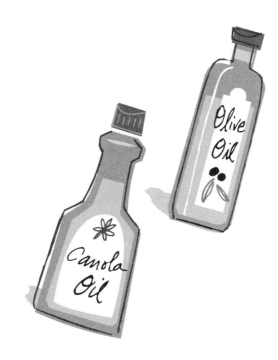

Crispy Cereal Treats

MAKES 12 SERVINGS

R ice Krispies Treats are Liz's Achilles' heel of desserts. She loved them as a kid, craved them during pregnancy, and even to this day finds it next to impossible to stop at just one! But they are
made with 6 cups of Rice Krispies, a bag of marshmallows, and 3 tablespoons of butter, so we decided to add our own healthy snap, crackle, and pop to this time-honored recipe. Now each treat is rich
in fiber and heart-healthy vitamin E, thanks to the high-fiber cereal and sunflower seeds. Don't be
concerned with the little bit of extra fat, because it's healthy fat from the sunflower seeds.

Moms Make It Over By . . .

- Using sunflower seeds for vitamins, minerals, phytonutrients,
  and fiber.
- Replacing some of the Rice Krispies with a whole grain cereal for
  added nutrients and fiber.
- Using canola oil in place of some of the butter to lower the
  saturated fat.

> 1 tablespoon butter
>
> 1 tablespoon canola oil
>
> One 10.5-ounce bag miniature marshmallows (about 4 cups)
>
> 1½ cups high-fiber cereal, such as Post 100% Bran or Trader Joe's
> High-Fiber Cereal
>
> 4 cups Rice Krispies cereal
>
> ½ cup roasted, shelled sunflower seeds, unsalted

1. Lightly oil or coat a 9 x 13-inch baking pan with nonstick cooking spray and set aside.

2. Heat the butter and oil in a large saucepan over low heat. When the butter is melted, add the
marshmallows and stir until completely melted. Remove from the heat.

3. Add the cereals and sunflower seeds and stir until well coated.

4. Press the mixture evenly into the baking pan using wax paper, a buttered spatula, or your buttered hands. Cool at room temperature and cut into 12 squares.

PREPARATION TIME: 10 MINUTES

Moms′ Kitchen Notes: Store leftovers in a plastic, airtight container.

	Before	After
Calories	150	170
Fat (g)	3	6
Saturated Fat (g)	2	1
Sodium (mg)	170	130
Carbohydrate (g)	31	30
Fiber (g)	0	4
Protein (g)	1	3

Sugar & Hyperactivity: Myth or Reality?

What makes children bounce off the walls: the birthday cake or the birthday party? The Halloween candy or the trick-or-treating? The goody bag treats or breaking open the piñata? Before you implicate sugar for your child's hyperactivity, consider that perhaps it's the event itself that brings on the behavior and not the sugar at all. There's no doubt that a small number of children are sensitive to sugar. But before you blacklist birthday cake, talk to your doctor for a bottom-line diagnosis.

Blueberry Snack Cake

MAKES 15 SERVINGS

Sour cream coffeecake may look innocent at first glance but the 1½ sticks of butter and 1½ cups of sour cream in some recipes make it a high-saturated-fat, high-calorie splurge with little redeeming nutritional value. We transformed this sweet cake into an irresistibly delicious snack. And by using blueberries, we added one of nature's most antioxidant-rich foods to your family's diet.

Moms Make It Over By ...

🥕 Adding blueberries for vitamins, minerals, phytonutrients, and fiber.

🥕 Using whole wheat flour and wheat germ for added nutrients and fiber.

🥕 Using canola oil to lower the saturated fat and increase the healthy omega-3 fats.

1¼ cups all-purpose flour

1¼ cups whole wheat flour

1 teaspoon baking powder

½ teaspoon baking soda

½ teaspoon salt

⅔ cup granulated sugar

⅓ cup canola oil

2 large eggs

1 teaspoon vanilla extract

One 6- or 8-ounce container lowfat lemon or vanilla yogurt

One 12-ounce bag frozen blueberries (about 2½ cups), or 1 pint fresh blueberries (about 2 cups)

TOPPING

½ cup quick-cooking oats

¼ cup packed brown sugar

¼ cup wheat germ

2 tablespoons canola oil

1 teaspoon ground cinnamon

1. Preheat the oven to 375°F.

2. Lightly oil or coat a 9 x 13-inch baking pan with nonstick cooking spray and set aside.

3. Whisk together the all-purpose flour, whole wheat flour, baking powder, baking soda, and salt in a medium bowl.

4. Meanwhile, add the sugar and oil to a large bowl and beat on medium speed until well blended, 1 minute. Scrape down the sides of the bowl if necessary.

5. Add the eggs and vanilla and continue to beat until smooth. Add the yogurt and beat until blended.

6. At low speed, gradually beat in the flour mixture until just combined. Gently stir in the blueberries.

7. Arrange the mixture evenly in the prepared pan and set aside.

8. To make the topping, combine the oats, brown sugar, wheat germ, oil, and cinnamon in a small bowl until the dry ingredients are moistened. Sprinkle evenly over the uncooked cake.

9. Bake for 45 to 50 minutes or until a toothpick inserted in the center comes out clean. Transfer the pan to a wire rack and cool for 10 minutes before slicing.

PREPARATION TIME: 20 MINUTES
COOKING TIME: 50 MINUTES

	Before	After
Calories	360	240
Fat (g)	17	9
Saturated Fat (g)	9	1
Sodium (mg)	390	170
Carbohydrate (g)	49	37
Fiber (g)	<1	3
Protein (g)	5	6

Moms' Kitchen Notes: Serve with a small scoop of frozen lowfat vanilla yogurt.

Brownie Mix Makeover

MAKES 20 SQUARES

When your kids get home from school and beg you to make brownies, what do you do? Do you grab for a boxed brownie mix? If you do, please don't feel guilty. We all do it from time to time because honestly, what could be easier? But unbeknownst to a lot of moms, most of those mixes contain hydrogenated oils. While eating a small amount of trans fats isn't the end of the world, we figured you'd appreciate a recipe that started with a trans-free brownie mix . . . so here goes.

Moms Make It Over By . . .

- Adding banana and wheat germ for vitamins, minerals, phytonutrients, and fiber.
- Using a brownie mix without hydrogenated oils to eliminate the trans fats.

> One 13.7-ounce box No Pudge! Fudge Brownie Mix
> ⅔ cup lowfat vanilla yogurt
> ½ cup wheat germ
> 1 ripe banana, mashed (about ½ cup)
> 2 large eggs, beaten

1. Preheat the oven to 350°F.
2. Lightly oil or coat a 7 x 11-inch baking pan with nonstick cooking spray and set aside.
3. Place the brownie mix, yogurt, wheat germ, banana, and eggs in a large bowl and beat with a spoon until the dry mix is moistened and the ingredients are well combined, about 2 minutes.
4. Spread the batter evenly into the prepared pan and bake for about 35 minutes, or until a toothpick inserted in the center comes out clean.
5. Transfer the pan to a rack and cool for 10 minutes before slicing.

PREPARATION TIME: 10 MINUTES
COOKING TIME: 35 MINUTES

	Before	After
Calories	230	100
Fat (g)	12	1
Saturated Fat (g)	1.5	0
Sodium (mg)	110	80
Carbohydrate (g)	28	20
Fiber (g)	0	1
Protein (g)	2	4

I-Can't-Believe-It's Bread Pudding

MAKES 8 SERVINGS

Bread pudding is simple and scrumptious. Most recipes call for just white bread, milk, eggs, and sugar. When we thought about the recipe, a lightbulb went on: What if we switched from white bread to something a bit healthier? To test our idea, we switched to a whole grain oat bread and the results were just as yummy.

Moms Make It Over by ...

- Using 1% lowfat milk to lower the saturated fat and calories.
- Switching to oat bread for added nutrients and fiber.

1¼ cups 1% lowfat milk

4 large eggs

½ cup sugar

1 teaspoon vanilla extract

7 slices whole grain oat bread, cut into ¾-inch cubes (about 6 cups)

¼ cup mini chocolate chips

1. Preheat the oven to 350°F.

2. Lightly oil or coat an 8 x 8-inch baking pan with nonstick cooking spray and set aside.

3. Whisk together the milk, eggs, sugar, and vanilla in a large bowl. Stir in the bread cubes and chocolate chips and mix well. Let stand at room temperature for 10 minutes. Stir occasionally to make sure all the bread is covered with the egg mixture.

4. Arrange the mixture evenly in the prepared pan and bake for 30 to 35 minutes, or until puffed and set.

5. Transfer the pan to a wire rack and cool for 5 minutes before slicing.

	Before	After
Calories	330	190
Fat (g)	14	6
Saturated Fat (g)	7	2
Sodium (mg)	410	160
Carbohydrate (g)	44	29
Fiber (g)	<1	2
Protein (g)	8	7

PREPARATION IME: 10 MINUTES
COOKING TIME: 35 MINUTES

Nut Sense

We recently ran across a bestselling low-fat cookbook published in the mid-1990s and noticed a so-called healthy recipe for brownies. For this particular recipe, we were shocked to see that the author purposely eliminated the nuts. Our reaction: Shame on you!

Nuts are ideal additions to baked goods because they impart a rich flavor and texture. They're also a good source of fiber, protein, antioxidants, and heart-healthy fats, namely monounsaturated and polyunsaturated fats. Eating just a small handful of nuts each day has been shown to lower cholesterol levels . . . an appetizing fact for people who once thought nuts were taboo. The following nuts are some of our favorites. Not only do they add a huge kick to many of our recipes, all are low in saturated fat.

WHAT'S IN A HANDFUL: $\frac{1}{4}$ cup (1 ounce)

NUT	CALORIES	PROTEIN (G)	FIBER (G)	TOTAL FAT (G)	SATURATED FAT (G)	MONOUNSATURATED FAT (G)	POLYUNSATURATED FAT (G)
Walnuts	180	4	2	18	1.5	2.5	13
Pecans	190	3	3	20	2	11.5	6.5
Almonds	160	6	3	14	1	9	4
Peanuts*	160	7	2.5	14	2	7	4.5

*Peanuts are actually a legume, a member of the same plant species as beans, peas, and soybeans.

Chocolate-Dipped Strawberries

MAKES 5 SERVINGS

What desserts do your kids ask for after dinner? Ice cream is at the top of our children's list. But ice cream, especially the super-rich kind, can have as much as half a day's worth of saturated fat in just one small bowl. A healthier and equally scrumptious option is our Chocolate-Dipped Strawberries. It's one of the easiest ways in the world to get your children to eat more fruit.

Moms Make It Over By . . .

🍓 Using strawberries for vitamins, minerals, phytonutrients, and fiber.

One 16-ounce carton fresh strawberries
½ cup semisweet mini chocolate chips

1. Remove the stems from the strawberries. Wash the berries under cold water and dry well with paper towels. Set aside.

2. Place the chocolate chips in a microwave-safe bowl and microwave on high for 30 seconds. Stir well and repeat 2 to 3 more times, just until the chips are melted. Do not overheat.

3. Divide the melted chocolate into small individual bowls. Let each family member dip their own strawberries (double dipping allowed!).

PREPARATION TIME: 10 MINUTES

	Before	After
Calories	300	110
Fat (g)	16	6
Saturated Fat (g)	10	3
Sodium (mg)	95	0
Carbohydrate (g)	34	17
Fiber (g)	0	3
Protein (g)	5	1

Moms' Kitchen Notes: Don't stop at strawberries. Pineapple, cantaloupe, and bananas are just as irresistible when paired with chocolate.

Apple & Pear Crisp

MAKES 8 TO 10 SERVINGS

Nothing could be more old-fashioned and homey than a cobbler, crisp, crumble, or buckle. Made with various types of fruit on the bottom and either a biscuit crust or a buttery mixture of flour and oats on the top, they're an easy way to slip more fruit into the diet. But given all the butter in a lot of these traditional desserts, the saturated fat can quickly add up. For that reason alone, we modernized the classic topping with better nutrition in mind.

Moms Make It Over By . . .

- Including wheat germ for vitamins, minerals, phytonutrients, and fiber.
- Using walnuts for added nutrients and healthy omega-3 fats.
- Using a small amount of canola oil versus a lot of butter to lower the saturated fat and calories.

3 to 4 large firm, ripe pears, peeled and cut into ¼-inch slices

3 to 4 large firm, tart apples, peeled and cut into ⅛-inch slices

2 tablespoons bottled or fresh lemon juice

½ cup raisins

2 tablespoons granulated sugar

2 tablespoons whole wheat flour

1 teaspoon ground cinnamon

TOPPING

½ cup quick-cooking oats

½ cup walnuts, finely chopped

⅓ cup packed brown sugar

⅓ cup wheat germ

½ teaspoon ground cinnamon

1 large egg, beaten

2 tablespoons canola oil

1. Preheat the oven to 350°F.

2. Combine the pears, apples, lemon juice, raisins, granulated sugar, whole wheat flour, and cinnamon in a large bowl and stir gently.

3. Transfer the fruit mixture to a 7 x 11-inch baking pan and set aside.

4. To make the topping, combine the oats, walnuts, brown sugar, wheat germ, cinnamon, egg, and oil in a medium bowl and mix well. Spread evenly over the fruit mixture.

5. Bake for 40 minutes, or until the fruit bubbles and the top turns golden brown.

PREPARATION TIME: 30 MINUTES
COOKING TIME: 40 MINUTES

	Before	After
Calories	340	270
Fat (g)	13	10
Saturated Fat (g)	8	1
Sodium (mg)	300	15
Carbohydrate (g)	57	46
Fiber (g)	6	6
Protein (g)	2	5

Moms' Kitchen Notes: Serve à la mode with lowfat frozen yogurt.

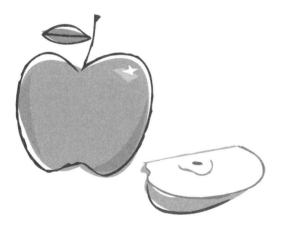

Carrot Cake with Lemony Glaze

MAKES 15 SERVINGS

With a name like carrot cake, it's got to be good for you, right? Well, even though it's loaded with shredded carrots, the buttery cream cheese frosting and the rich batter in many recipes can push the saturated fat and calories into the red zone. In fact, a slice of carrot cake can be even more decadent than a slice of chocolate layer cake. Carrot cake goes from a C-minus to an A-plus with our easy makeover.

Moms Make It Over By . . .

- Adding pineapple for vitamins, minerals, phytonutrients, and fiber.
- Using pecans for added nutrients and heart-healthy monounsaturated fats.
- Using canola oil to lower the saturated fat and increase the healthy omega-3 fats.
- Creating a light glaze to reduce the sugar and calories.

1 cup all-purpose flour

1 cup whole wheat flour

¼ cup wheat germ

2 teaspoons ground cinnamon

1 teaspoon baking powder

½ teaspoon baking soda

¼ teaspoon salt

1 cup granulated sugar

½ cup canola oil

3 large eggs

1 teaspoon vanilla extract

4 large carrots, shredded (about 4 cups)

One 8-ounce can crushed pineapple in its own juice, well drained

1 cup pecans, finely chopped

GLAZE

½ cup confectioners' sugar

2 tablespoons bottled or fresh lemon juice

1. Preheat the oven to 375°F.

2. Lightly oil or coat a 9 x 13-inch baking pan with nonstick cooking spray and set aside.

3. Whisk together the all-purpose flour, whole wheat flour, wheat germ, cinnamon, baking powder, baking soda, and salt in a medium bowl.

4. Combine the sugar and oil in a large bowl and beat on medium speed until well blended, 1 minute. Add the eggs and vanilla and continue to beat until smooth. Scrape down the sides of the bowl if necessary.

5. At low speed, gradually beat in the flour mixture until just combined. Add the carrots, pineapple, and pecans and stir to combine.

6. Spread the mixture evenly into the prepared pan. Bake about 35 minutes, or until a toothpick inserted in the center of the cake comes out clean.

7. While the cake is cooling, prepare the glaze by whisking together the powdered sugar and lemon juice in a small bowl until smooth. Drizzle over the warm cake.

PREPARATION TIME: 35 MINUTES
COOKING TIME: 35 MINUTES

	Before	After
Calories	590	290
Fat (g)	32	15
Saturated Fat (g)	8	1.5
Sodium (mg)	280	135
Carbohydrate (g)	73	37
Fiber (g)	2	3
Protein (g)	6	5

Moms' Kitchen Notes: To speed things up a bit, use 3 or 4 cups preshredded carrots. If the shreds are long, chop them up a bit.

Banana Chocolate Chip Muffins

MAKES 12 MUFFINS

When most people hear the word "muffin," they think "healthy." When we hear the word, however, we think "donut." The original recipe for Banana Chocolate Chip Muffins came from Liz's neighbor, who wanted to cut the 2 sticks of butter from her children's favorite after-school treat without changing the flavor too dramatically. What we came up with sets a good example for what a muffin should be!

Moms Make It Over By . . .

- Using canola oil versus butter to lower the saturated fat and increase the healthy omega-3 fats.
- Including whole wheat flour and wheat germ for added nutrients and fiber.

> 1 cup all-purpose flour
> ½ cup whole wheat flour
> ¼ cup wheat germ
> 2 teaspoons baking powder
> ¼ teaspoon salt
> 2 ripe bananas, mashed (about 1 cup)
> 2 large eggs, beaten
> ½ cup packed brown sugar
> ⅓ cup canola oil
> ⅓ cup 1% lowfat milk
> 1 teaspoon vanilla
> ½ cup mini chocolate chips

1. Preheat the oven to 350°F.

2. Lightly oil or coat 12 muffin cups with nonstick cooking spray and set aside.

3. Whisk together the all-purpose flour, whole wheat flour, wheat germ, baking powder, and salt in a large bowl.

4. Combine the bananas, eggs, sugar, oil, milk, and vanilla in a medium bowl and stir until well blended.

5. Pour the liquid ingredients over the dry ingredients and stir until just moistened. Stir in the chocolate chips.

6. Spoon the batter into the prepared muffin cups. Bake about 20 minutes, or until the muffins are light golden and a toothpick inserted in the center comes out clean.

7. Transfer the pan to a wire rack and cool for 5 minutes. Remove the muffins and cool an additional 5 minutes before serving.

PREPARATION TIME: 20 MINUTES
COOKING TIME: 20 MINUTES

	Before	After
Calories	290	220
Fat (g)	14	10
Saturated Fat (g)	9	2
Sodium (mg)	240	140
Carbohydrate (g)	39	31
Fiber (g)	1	2
Protein (g)	3	4

Moms' Kitchen Notes: Let the kids help by coating the muffin cups and stirring in the chocolate chips.

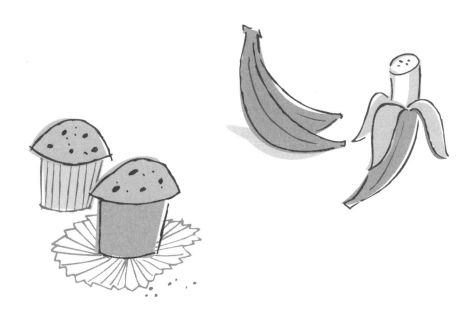

Better-Than-Store-Bought "Jell-O"

MAKES 6 SERVINGS

Every year, 300 million boxes of Jell-O are sold in the United States alone and it's easy to see why. Kids love its jiggly, wiggly, squish-in-your-mouth appeal. What we don't particularly love about this all-American dessert, however, are the artificial colors and flavors that come packed in every little box. Our solution: making a Jell-O-like dessert from scratch. Our makeover takes about 3 extra minutes to prepare and comes with a few extra nutrients to boot, including calcium and vitamin C.

Moms Make It Over By . . .

- Adding Mandarin oranges for vitamins, minerals, and phytonutrients.
- Switching to unflavored gelatin to eliminate the artificial flavors and colors.
- Using calcium-fortified orange juice for vitamin C and calcium.

> **One 11-ounce can Mandarin oranges, drained**
>
> **1 packet unflavored gelatin (1 tablespoon)**
>
> **½ cup boiling water**
>
> **¼ cup sugar**
>
> **⅛ teaspoon salt**
>
> **1½ cups calcium-fortified orange juice**

1. Divide the Mandarin oranges evenly between 6 custard cups or small bowls and set aside.

2. Combine the gelatin with ¼ cup cold water in a medium bowl and let soften, 3 minutes.

3. Add the boiling water, sugar, and salt and stir until the sugar dissolves. Add the orange juice to the gelatin mixture, stir, and divide evenly among the custard cups.

4. Chill until the liquid sets, 2 to 3 hours.

PREPARATION TIME: **10 MINUTES**

CHILL TIME: **2 TO 3 HOURS**

	Before	After
Calories	80	70
Fat (g)	0	0
Saturated Fat (g)	0	0
Sodium (mg)	40	55
Carbohydrate (g)	19	17
Fiber (g)	0	0
Protein (g)	2	1

Moms' Kitchen Notes: For a "gelatin creamsicle," replace ½ cup of the orange juice with ½ cup lowfat vanilla yogurt.

Index

Join the Club

As you learned in the introduction to *The Moms' Guide to Meal Makeovers,* your meal makeover journey need not begin and end with this book. By visiting our website, www.mealmakeovermoms.com, you'll have an opportunity to join the Meal Makeover Moms' Club. As a member, you'll be able to enjoy the following benefits:

- A monthly newsletter with food and nutrition news and our latest makeover recipes
- An opportunity to submit your favorite family recipes for a healthy makeover
- Information on new food products that we consider the Best of the Bunch
- A place where your questions and concerns about feeding children will be answered by the Meal Makeover Moms themselves
- A chance to create your own customized supermarket shopping list
- Links to online bookstores
- And much much more

We look forward to hearing from you!

Liz & Janice